praise for EYI

"A wonderful true story that
feelings...from frustration to reuc...
Sebastian's verbal visual processing is a fascinating case that is transforming our understanding of CVI. A must-read for any family facing the challenges of raising a child with any disability."
- *Dr. Lotfi Merabet, director of the Harvard CVI Neuroplasticity research study, associate scientist at Massachusetts Eye and Ear, and associate professor of ophthalmology at Harvard Medical School*

"In her inaugural book, Duesing takes us on an intimate journey through her family's struggle in obtaining a diagnosis and the necessary services for their son with cerebral/cortical visual impairments (CVI). Their experience provides compelling evidence for the need to better understand the brain changes associated with CVI and how these impact how one views the world."
- *Corinna Bauer, PhD., investigator at the Massachusetts Eye and Ear, and instructor of ophthalmology at Harvard Medical School*

"The touching story of a bright teenager with undiagnosed and untreated cerebral visual impairments and his mother's struggle to have these invisible disorders recognized. This story is as important to patients and their families as it is to the educational and medical institutions. Cerebral visual impairments need to be better known, better diagnosed, better managed, and this book will certainly contribute to that."
- *Dr. Sylvie Chokron, director of research, Unit of Vision and Cognition at La Fondation Rothschild, Paris, France*

"An amazing story that left me both inspired and intrigued. Stephanie Duesing relates the far-reaching implications of the complex and widely misunderstood diagnosis of cerebral visual impairment. After reading of this family's honest and engaging perspective on their path to understanding, professionals will be compelled towards conscientious reflection and consideration of the experiences offered by parents and children."
- *Mindy S. Ely, PhD., assistant professor of low vision/blindness programs and EL VISTA project co-coordinator, Illinois State University*

"Stephanie Duesing's compelling new book, *Eyeless Mind*, is as warm and humorous as it is insightful and sometimes distressing. The author deftly weaves her remembrances of her difficult childhood through the narrative of her quest to find the correct diagnosis for her gifted son, Sebastian. A must read and an epic love letter to the significance of music and art education for children."
- *Alexandra Patsavas, Music Producer/Soundtrack Producer, Credits including The O.C., Mad Men, Grey's Anatomy, "The Twilight Series," Supernatural, and Riverdale*

"A harrowing, heartbreaking, and inspiring tale of mother and son as they find their way through personal and professional forms of tunnel vision. A testament to the power of love and adaptation, and to the importance of seeing - and feeling seen."
- *Meg Jay, PhD., author of Supernormal and The Defining Decade*

"Do you ever feel like someone is looking at you—even speaking to you, but they don't really see you? Once in a great while, a family story becomes more—much more. This is just such a story—one that teaches the importance of trusting your gut and defending the truth.

"It is acceptable for doctors not to know everything, but it is not acceptable for doctors to believe that they do. It is not acceptable for a doctor to refuse to see and hear you as you explain what you know to be true.

"Stephanie's story is one of undying love for her son—the story of a seemingly endless journey to find the truth in a world where the truth only lies in a medical journal. It is proof positive that you must stop and wait to be seen—to be heard—before you can tell your story.

"*Eyeless Mind* is a story worth reading—a moving account of motherly love founded on the belief that God's truth always wins in the end. Let this story give you strength when medical issues plague you and you know in your heart what medical professionals refuse to accept.

"'Even when you have never seen the air we breathe or the wind that moves the largest oak tree, do you need proof that it exists?'"
- *Terry Stafford, award-winning author of Strings of Faith and the Brandon McStocker Series*

"*Eyeless Mind* is a fascinating portrait of an extraordinary American family. Moving, personal, and, at times, humorous, Duesing draws the reader in to experience a major medical discovery right along with her—and then we all witness the power of the arts to heal."
- *John Hildreth, teacher, actor and director*

"The importance of telling the story of Sebastian Duesing and his parents' journey in seeking a diagnosis and understanding of a specific visual processing condition cannot be minimized. It is a story of parental perseverance in spite of incredulity of both medical and educational professionals. This letter of endorsement is from the perspective of an educator in the field of visual impairments, the very discipline that has a major responsibility in determining vision-related services provided by the school. It is also a story of educational disbelief, neglect, and refusal to provide services by all involved school personnel.

"One of the major purposes of education is to promote critical thinking and problem-solving skills in learners. It appears that neither were employed when it came to selecting assessment instruments to examine Sebastian's functional use of vision and in interpreting the results. Most of the assessment tools were totally inappropriate and, more seriously, administered by professionals ill-equipped to go beyond the formulas dictated by the chosen instruments.

"It should be noted that Sebastian is not the only student who has suffered from the fate he endured. He is, however, the most unusual and, to date, the only one identified with verbal-visual processing dysfunction. Hopefully, this book will result in some changes for both pre-service and in-service training. Although it is important to introduce both TVI and O&M learners to varying assessment tools and methods of instruction, perhaps the most important skill to impart is being open to idea that the "flat world" may not be flat, the impossible may be possible, and the incredible may be credible. This is what I learned from Sebastian Duesing."
- Mary T. Morse, PhD., special education consultant for students with multiple disabilities and/or deafblindness

EYELESS MIND

A Memoir about Seeing and Being Seen

Stephanie Duesing

atmosphere press

Published by Atmosphere Press

Cover art and additional art by Sebastian Duesing
Cover design by Nick Courtright
Author photo by Brian McConkey

Some names and identifying details have been changed to protect the privacy of individuals and some dialogue has been reconstructed from memory.

Identifiers:
LCCN: 2019920906
ISBN: 978-1-64746-092-1 (paperback)
ISBN: 978-1-64746-094-5 (ebook)

Eyeless Mind: A Memoir about Seeing and Being Seen
2020, Stephanie L. Duesing

atmospherepress.com

To Lukas Franck:
You are your father's greatest work.

Author's Note

This book is a true story that deals with abuse and medical malpractice. All of the stories within it are true and told without exaggeration to the best of my ability. I have concealed the identities of some wonderful people for privacy reasons, and I have concealed the identities, appearances, and the locations of all of the doctors who failed us for legal reasons. We share our story in the hopes that no other family experiences what we experienced. I have thirty-six single spaced typed pages of documentation of our medical journey, and every quote of significance said by a doctor in this book is truly a quote. Other conversations or minor parts of conversations are reconstructed from memory. I am a survivor of life-threatening child abuse and I have lived openly as such since the summer of 2001. All of the stories about the abuse I experienced from my mother were shared with my therapist over a two-year period beginning that summer, as well as with my husband Eric Duesing, and my many good friends. My mother's abusive behavior was so open and pervasive that I have multiple witnesses, including my husband and friends from high school, one of whom reported what she saw to a trusted adult. She says that she is "haunted" by what she saw.

ACT ONE

One-Woman Show

"The willow which bends to the tempest, often escapes better than the oak which resists it, and so in great calamities, it sometimes happens that light and frivolous spirits recover their elasticity and presence of mind sooner than those of a loftier character." - Albert Schweitzer

"Blindness is just another way of seeing." - Dr. Lotfi Merabet, director of the Harvard CVI Neuroplasticity research study, associate scientist at Massachusetts Eye and Ear, and associate professor of ophthalmology at Harvard Medical School

I abandoned Sebastian 540 times between the ages of three and six, minus that week in February I kept him home when my mom died. There was also the week when he had strep, and assorted other days when he was under the weather. Sebastian often had an upset tummy in the mornings. "Mama, my tummy hurts," was his morning refrain. Let's say another ten days. That comes to about 520 times.

I didn't mean to abandon him. I would never intentionally abandon any living creature, especially my own child. I did intentionally dump my mom, though. Well, we abandoned each other, really. It's a different thing, abandoning a child. Sebastian cried every time I walked off and left him. Honestly, it was concerning, frustrating, and totally mystifying at the time. I wonder how things would have been different for Sebastian and myself without that universe of pain that threatened to crush us like new stars in a nebula.

My mom, though, oh, that's complicated. I'm certain she cried when I abandoned her. Her brief stint in modeling school and one part in a community theater play sometime in the early 1960s had prepared her surprisingly well for a life of drama. She had played Woman with a Toothache in one forgotten production. I can still picture the old black-and-white photo of her with the cast; her jaw bound up with a white bandage and knotted at the top of her head. The black cat eyeglasses glinted sharply in the hammock of white fabric between chin and hairline, not really concealing her embarrassment at being "caught on film in such a get-up."

The modeling school photo is harder to process, but the fragility is there if you look. In that photo, she poses glamorously with her feet stacked properly and one hip cocked. She paid attention in class to the angle of the toes and the turn of the hip. She models a sensible brown winter woolen suit. You can sense the disappointment that after all these classes on deportment and posture, she's been assigned a thick and dumpy clot of wool for the final show.

"It's nothing like the elegant black satin evening gown with the plunging décolletage that was featured on the modeling school's *Toronto Sun* advertisement," she said.

The best part of this photo is the handwritten note in black ink across the corner. Her ordinarily small and neat penmanship is a loud and outraged cursive.

"*Where did they get that hat?*"

I wonder that, too. It was spectacularly ugly, heavy and helmet-like, falling low across the forehead. It looked almost as if a feed bucket tipped over in the barn and landed with a sucking plop there on her head.

Mom looks less embarrassed in this photo than in the theater shot, but there's a sadness, maybe, and a defensiveness lingering beneath the fragile swagger. I can see through the confident posture, the hand on the hip, and it's there in the tilt of the chin and the forced smile. It's the defiant begging quality of a woman desperate for approval. She is trying to act.

Devotees of Michael Shurtleff would recognize the action: To Impress! But the subtext is there too, in the eyes, and it says, "I'm not good enough, and I never will be." My mom was a woman with fabulous dreams that were constantly disappointed by reality. I wonder if that day at modeling school was the moment she began to create her own play. It was a one-woman show where she got all the best roles.

"Ingenue and bride are boring, everyone knows that," she said.

She played those parts, and the part of the long-suffering wife, but it was that most sought-after role of hero that she wanted so badly to play. She imagined herself dashing down her enemy and vanquishing all who challenged her authoritarian impulses. In the doing, she unknowingly became a method actor. She became the role most cherished by all female actors. That desire for revenge, to hurt and punish all who betrayed her innocence as a girl, transformed her Don Quixote into the spying, plotting witch. She went into the woods, and it was a transformation that was lost on her completely.

My mother only ever saw herself as a Don Quixote, and in some way, I suppose she was. But the only fair princess she could find the inclination to protect was herself as Magdalena. Mom played all the roles, but she never took curtain calls for her best ones.

I am certain that she cried when I left her. I can picture her with her hands over her face, shoulders shaking. Poorly mimicked sadness and fake cries of sorrow puff through her hands, artificial, with the fingers carefully spread to conceal the lack of tears. I remember that at times like this, her eyes were watchful, not tearful. She would peek between her fingers when she thought no one was looking to gauge the effect of her performance. Both eyes and mouth would be absurdly rounded in mock grief and pretend innocence. A car accident had blinded one of her eyes, but both could be awfully soulless for a woman who had had a near-death experience.

The official story was that Mom flipped her VW Beetle on a windy Canadian highway. It was a huge pothole, she told us. A young, buxom blonde, Mom was a ski bunny for Winterfest sometime in the late 1950s or early 1960s. She was a bunny before there were Bunnies. She was a gifted and dedicated teacher who loved to sing, though she had no formal musical training. She was spending the summer in Deep River as a hotel chambermaid to earn some extra cash. There were picnics at the lake and bonfires in the evening. Deep River was the place to go for young people to meet—and meet they did. Mom met my dad, and then met her pothole as she headed home to Pickering. They had one dance before she almost died.

I try to imagine the screams and flames, the tangled wreck of twisted steel, but I'm not good with gore. My inner watcher is revolted and shies away. It peeks with horror at these old tales, remembering the scent of her Chanel No. 5 body powder as she sat in bra and panties on the king-size bed in San Jose. Mom told the story to us kids as she put her makeup on before she finished dressing. The smell of talcum and Chanel No. 5 was sickly sweet, absurdly infantile, and incongruous with her large breasts and plus-size figure.

After the accident, Mom was in a body cast for a year. Skin grafts made cheesy pizza of her back and shoulders. I remember the silken and cool texture of the scar tissue on her left arm. It was always a few degrees cooler than the healthy skin beside it. Her left foot was crushed, and though it healed, it healed stiff and perfectly flat on the bottom. Her gait was uneven and clumping. The failed model who before the accident wore three-inch heels daily to teach in was forever after shod like a Clydesdale.

She told us a piece of cartilage broke loose and lodged in the artery that fed the optic nerve, and it cut off the blood to her left eye. I can see in my imagination the wild white mote balanced behind her eye like a tiny funerary coin. Instead of weighing down the lids of the dead, this tiny coin sparks questions: What do the dead see? What, really, do the living see? I still wonder where exactly the line between the two is drawn.

It's amazing that she lived. Only now, as an adult, do I begin to comprehend the agony of what she survived. I remember asking her what it was like to almost die. She saw a light, she told us, a bright light, and there was a voice that urged her to go back. And so she did, for her Act Two.

This next part of the story is blurry for me; I heard it only once, when I was young. The only photo of my mother in which she looks somewhat natural is her cheesecake pinup that she had done before her wedding. In the picture she is kneeling, angled to the side. She wears a body-fitting black turtleneck, and the angle favors the curve of her youthful breasts.

"The photographer told me to take off my skirt," she said. The long, shapely legs, elegant in black hosiery, are tucked beneath her, her small bottom curving upwards from the cup of the soles of her feet. She is radiant. The blonde hair is perfectly coiffed in her signature updo, and the smile is fun and optimistic instead of sultry. But it's the eyes again that throw me off. I saw this photo for the first time when I was a child, but it wasn't until after she passed away that I realized the photo was scandalous for its time.

My mom married my dad in a civil ceremony. In the photos, he is tall, dark, and handsome with a tennis player's lanky physique. Mom designed her dress after Jackie Kennedy's style, with the pencil skirt and silk jacket with large self-covered fabric buttons. She wore a tiny round tiara over her chignon, and her heavy black cat eyeglasses dominate her lovely face in the wedding pictures. Years later she would tell me of her mother's wedding gift to her. As my mother arrived at the courthouse to be married, Grandma Slater pursed her lips and softly hissed, in her whispery English accent, "My friend said that I'm still prettier than you are."

As newlyweds, my parents traveled to Boston. Dad began his doctorate at MIT while my mother began a different type of performance career. She found a job teaching at an exclusive private school and continued to work even after her first baby was born in the summer of 1966. The downstairs neighbors watched the baby while Mom kept the income coming in. My sister slept in a drawer, and my mom used a board beneath the cushions of the sofa to abate the sag. She hosted a dinner party with some physics department bigwigs, and I think it was the department head who sat and broke the sofa. My mother was embarrassed about that all her life.

Her teaching was more successful than her dinner parties. She told me she taught one of President Gerald Ford's children, although I don't know which one. They gave her a Christmas ornament in thanks: an Oscar. Every year at Christmastime I'd unpack the ornaments to find the gleaming fish. The pink-and-purple-sequined scales were prickly and oddly lifelike, if something can be lifelike in death.

Once at a Chinese restaurant, my mother ordered fish. It arrived, head and all, with the gaping mouth and large, flat unseeing eyes that stared in shock around the dining table. I'm sure my own eyes stared right back in horror and fascination. How could anyone eat something with eyes that watched you as you ate it? The accusatory eyes looked exactly like its fabric cousin's that swam through streams of glowing, scented needles instead of rivers of silty water.

Every Christmas that cold, dead white sequin eye looked down upon us. We were atheists who celebrated our own versions of Christmas and Easter. We had a children's Bible, but the lessons were, "These are only fairy tales for people who fear death," and "Scientists don't believe in things they cannot prove." Our oscar supervised the cold exchange of gifts.

Although she couldn't see out of one, both of my mom's eyes communicated more than she wished. Both eyes were mobile and expressive. They were large and blue, and in photos she stretched them wide as she smiled. It was an old trick from her modeling classes, to make the eyes look larger. In practice, it gave her photos a stressed and anxious look.

But I remember her eyes; my inner watcher sees those eyes. I remember them dancing with unconcealed glee, or worse, dry and watchful, searching for her audience's reaction. I can still see her lips pout in an imitation of a child's sulk, the finger-shadowed orbs first a caricature of grief and hurt, and then, triumph! She's won! They believe her! The fake sobs give way to delicate little sniffs as she tucks her chin to look up at her fans through fluttering eyelashes, never realizing that no one believes—they just don't care.

I can still see her standing in the kitchen of our split-level ranch in Darien, Illinois, the early evening light softly bathing her. I'm hiding my too-tall four-year-old self in the shadow behind the black leather easy chair in the family room. The black faux leather is stained on the headrest from men's pomade. I can see the kitchen table—a card table—behind her with a plastic top and the four metal folding chairs around it. My baby brother's yellow plastic highchair is in the corner. She's on the phone again.

"It was so scary," she says into the receiver. "How could this have happened? It was such a terrible accident."

She pauses and takes a drag from her Salem Light.

"Well, now the neighbors are talking about it, and it's not my fault. After all, I was so worried!"

Oh, yes. She was worried all right.

Not worried enough to show up on my first day of kindergarten at pickup time. Not worried enough to call the school and ask them to hold me in the office until she got there, flustered and embarrassed. Not worried enough to ask a neighbor for help, or to call a babysitter to watch my baby brother while he napped.

In my mind's eye, I can still see her, babbling on and on into the phone. Sometimes she blames the washing machine repairman. Other times she says that the pipe burst in the basement, but there was never any water damage. It was the plumber's fault on those days. It's hard for her to keep the details straight as she drinks cold black coffee and chain smokes, rehashing the tale to her Toronto family and then her friend in Idaho.

Every time she tells a new version of the tale, for two weeks I hear those words: "I was *so* worried." She loves to drawl out her vowels, as though the extra sounds make up for the lack of a credible story. Her big blue eyes are extremely serious, as though the listener can see through the telephone wires, into the phone box in the kitchen, through the long spiraling wire, and out the handset to examine the sincerity of her expression. She was worried, all right. She was worried she'd get caught.

I come by my child abandonment skills rightfully.

So, I abandoned Sebastian too. What did we decide? Five hundred and forty times, minus the week my mom died, or thereabouts. Then there was the week of first grade he missed when he had strep, and the many days when he had a low-grade fever but no obvious loss of the rippling spring of continuous movement that followed him everywhere as he played. Pneumonia in second grade would finally bring him to the couch for several scary and watchful days, but until then, he romped through every fever and cold.

I remember him that late May day as a first grader as he pirouetted through the kitchen, leaped into the dining room, and disappeared under the dining room table, announcing, "I'm Darry, King of the Fairies and Professor of Defense Against the Dark Arts. You can't see me!"

He was right. I didn't see him for ten more years. No matter how many times I abandoned him, I didn't see him. I think my eyes were blind. I take comfort in knowing that he was, indeed, invisible. His camouflage was woven out of words.

I could not see him. I tried. I really did. But no one saw him, just as no one saw me abandon him, even though I left him, again and again, to fend for himself alone in this world without a soul to guide his steps. I, who know intimately the shrieking fear of walking alone down unknown roads, every hair stiff as needles, whispering desperately, "Mommy! Mommy, where are you?" Some deep ancient instinct kept me from screaming; some prehistoric wisdom knew that to advertise my aloneness too loudly could invite further nightmares. Me. I abandoned my son.

I still try to imagine seeing right into his head, looking through Sebastian's eyes, like a grotesque inversion of the ancient marble statue Young Satyr with Mask. Age and Responsibility try vainly to comprehend the constant unfolding newness of this child's vision of the world.

Everyone saw his incredible beauty: the silky soft wisps of short blond hair and the perfection of the planes of his cheekbones. Fleeting dimples appeared with every rosebud smile, like a sprig of baby's breath perfuming his delight. And those eyes—those unknowable eyes. Sebastian's eyes are light. They are the perfect mid-china blue Duesing eyes that stun me with their symmetry, not at all like mine.

My left eye is smaller than the right, a source of vexation in every photo. Not that it matters, as I blink every time a camera flashes. They had to pull me aside at the DMV for a special session. I was holding up the line. Apparently, it's inconvenient to fellow citizens to have eyes that shy from the nuclear blasts of flash photography.

Sebastian's eyes are brilliant, a reflection of his mind, but opaque to my soul. His eyes missed nothing and everything. Light ran through those dark pupils and shimmered beneath the surface of his irises like star sapphires, their gentle cabochons polished by his sweep of light brown lashes.

Right now, my inner watcher sees those happy glimpses of his eyes as a first grader in late May. Sebastian had tied Magic Cabin play silks around his waist. Six feet of rainbow-colored silk murmured from his shoulders in a ripple of liquid first grader as he burst out from under the table. He flashed me a radiant dimpled smile before streaming off to do battle with Snape and Voldemort.

"Expelliarmus!"

We PTO ladies of Lincoln Elementary School were assembling the end-of-year scrapbook to memorialize the uncertain success of Sebastian's first year teacher, who was taking her skills to another district school. I was sympathetic, as I had once been a first-year teacher too. Sympathetic, and I was glad the year was over. I had looked forward to a morning with some adult conversation with the other ladies, but of course, Sebastian had strep. Now my attention was divided between these very nice ladies, a task I had no business doing, and this magnetic child.

I had been pressed into volunteering for the job of creating the scrapbook, but having no success at scrapbooking in general,

I had sent a desperate email invitation to the other classroom moms asking for assistance. It was a plea for help. There's nothing like the temptation of getting the cutest photos of your own child prominently featured in even the most mundane of projects to rally PTO moms. Come they did, and thank goodness, as I had purchased some $1,500 worth of Creative Memories scrapbooking supplies to make Sebastian's baby book and then discovered I had no aptitude for it.

I completed the first six months of his baby book while he was still a sweet milky-scented fuzz of warmth on my shoulder, little legs tucked up and that padded diapered bottom just a handful. My artistic pretensions were easy to indulge when he napped twice a day. I proudly finished Sebastian's baby book when he was three. I felt a sense of achievement; I had accomplished something important. I went through the photos while he was sleeping.

He was always such a good sleeper. We ate dinner with the blue-haired people at five o'clock, so we could get him to bed no later than six. Sebastian was an early riser. For two solid years, I was awakened by that precious small voice and gentle touch of tiny hands.

"Mama, I'm ready to play with you."

He woke me at 4:45 every morning like clockwork. No matter how much you love your child, there's nowhere to go and nothing to do with a toddler from 5 a.m. until 10 a.m. It was Sebastian and me, with my questionable artistic skills. I was outmatched. I gave birth to Albert Einstein's and Martha Stewart's love child, and I'm not either one.

There was never a child who loved to create more than Sebastian did. He was insatiable. We colored, drew, painted, and made popsicle-stick art with noodles and feathers. I gave up keeping his clothes clean when he painted. Once the first piece of paper had some color on it, nothing would do but to paint his own skin. So, he painted naked at the easel and in the bathtub.

"Look, Mama! I'm putting overalls on!" He laughed as he trailed blue bathtub finger paint up one beautifully muscled shoulder and down the other.

He was born an artist. That day when he was three and he wanted to help with his baby book, I handed him the acid-free stickers and gave him two pages of his own. They are still there, the silky fabric of the Snow White dress on its tiny wire hanger pressed against the page, and random Halloween-themed stickers scattered about. I love to linger over that page. I touch the yellow satin on the skirt, and I can still see Sebastian swinging in the backyard.

He wears his favorite outfit, a bright yellow fleece Carter's top with a bug on it and matching striped pants. He's been wearing this outfit every day now for a year, so it's eighty-seven degrees outside, and he's dressed in yellow fleece and long pants. I swelter uncomfortably in my cotton shorts and T-shirt as I push his small bottom to race toward the eye of the sun, and I comfort myself with the fact that at least his shirt is short sleeved now, and the pants are becoming floods. I sneak the favorite outfit into the laundry every night.

I tried to get Sebastian to wear other things for those two years. When he fell in love with the bug shirt, I went back to Carter's and bought similar shirts in other colors. But neither the dark purple ant shirt or the orange truck one was acceptable. I thought it was the bug that he loved, but it was the color. He wore nothing but yellow from head to toe for two years. He loved yellow.

The other purple and orange tops lay neglected in their drawer, a silent indictment. Why didn't I go back to the store sooner, before all the yellow ones were gone? I can still see him in this favorite costume. I see his small, perfect fists clutched around the chains of the swing.

"Red rover, red rover, send Sebastian right over!"

I give him a big push and catch his shining eyes as they meet mine. I dash past on his right, but not really giving the real Red Rover. He's too little for that. For now, he's delighted with the rhyme and the extra height. He's learning to pump. He's trying to propel himself by yanking the chains and finding the rhythm of the weightlessness. His rhythm is off but he's trying to fly. His blond hair flutters in the breeze and his gray shadow brushes the battered grass beneath the swing with every pass. My heart tugs as he leaves my reach and with every return it lifts, relieved. I am overwhelmed with love for him.

It's August. And tomorrow, I will abandon him.

Medea

"It's been said that more than 60% of human communication is nonverbal," I typed. It was the end of August 2016 and I was trying to get a jump on my September newsletter for my Musikgarten families. "Facial expressions, gestures, even subtle looks communicate meaning, with or without words."

The soft strains of the Largo movement of Bach's Trio Sonata in C minor played in the background, the haunting violin melody pulling my attention away from the task at hand. I took a sip of water and kept typing.

"Children who engage in music have opportunities to develop better social skills than those who don't," I typed, mentally thanking Dr. Dee Coulter, neuroscience educator, for what must have been the millionth time. I didn't need to read her work to know this fact, though her neuroscience of music Musikgarten packet was sitting right beside me. "Music, with its multicultural appeal, helps different people to bond together over shared experiences of its universal language."

My internal soundtrack annoyingly played "Ring Around the Rosie" over the Bach as I pictured the scene from my toddler class this morning. As I greeted my friend Katie Johnson, her girls Laynie and Harper started dancing. Katie was an artist with cut and color, and a dear friend who had listened to all my griefs and triumphs. When I opened my Musikgarten business, Katie was my first client. She brought two-year-old Laynie and her new baby, Harper. Laynie was something else.

On her very first trip to my home for class, Laynie opened up the screen door, let herself in, and said, "I'm here to sing songs with you." She was not yet two and speaking in full sentences. She reminded me of Sebastian at that age.

Today Laynie and Harper grabbed hands with Michael, who they met only last week, and danced around and around. Jamal joined in as soon as he walked in the door, and then observant Phoebe started dancing. Class hadn't even started yet and these little humans were singing in tune and dancing, making eye contact and interacting with unbridled joy. I saw the wonder in the parents' eyes, and the satisfaction.

"You are helping your child to develop better social skills by participating in daily music at home," I continued typing, thinking: *How do I say this? This is a sensitive subject and I know I write the world's longest newsletters for these busy young parents. How to be brief but honest? I have dads too, so this is for all of them.* I thought of what I had learned from Cathy Mathia and my other mentors at my Musikgarten training classes, and then continued.

"This month we will be learning lots of cheerful songs and games to encourage gross motor activity. As we learned in last month's news, tying actions to words is how toddlers learn vocabulary. That is why we sing about jumping while we jump, etc.," I re-explained.

Most of my parents were on board now with understanding how small children acquire language through movement, but it never hurts to remind them. *Now for the tough part,* I thought to myself, *and the major topic of this month's news.*

"However, there will be one minor lullaby and a song in Dorian mode, which is an old church mode that sounds similar to minor." I ran my hands through my hair and paused, considering. "These two songs express a longing, or a sadness."

I paused to take a sip of water before launching into the next part. I have only ever had one parent complain about this lovely, haunting lullaby, but her desire to have every single song sound happy had made me think. She may not be the only one with this mindset.

"Sometimes parents ask why we include an occasional sad-sounding song in the curriculum. The reason is simple. It is a deliberate choice on the part of the creators of the program." I paused again to consider my wording, and then I had it.

"Musikgarten was created to engage all parts of your child's development, including the social and emotional elements," I continued. "Your children will experience grief and loss sometime in their lives. As much as we try to protect them, they will experience the loss of a beloved pet, sometimes divorce, sometimes the death of grandparents, and even close friends leave when families have to relocate."

There we go. That's the right tone to take, I thought with satisfaction.

"Having songs to sing when one is sad helps children learn to understand and label their own feelings. At home, you can encourage this behavior. It will help them to process when they are frustrated or angry, too."

You will be grateful for this ability when you have a teenager like I do, I thought with amusement. Then I decided to type it. My families knew me and would get the joke. Sebastian was so easy, it was ridiculous.

I glanced at the Shaker clock on the old blue chest by the window. Everyone asked me if the battered deep-blue piece was from Pottery Barn, but the old walnut sideboard was authentically distressed. My mom bought it at the Salvation Army in Boston fifty years ago and then antiqued it blue. I still remember seeing my little brother riding his red trike right into it when it was sitting in the driveway in San Jose, waiting by the moving van. The mark was still there in the trim around the door. We leave impressions as we go through life, intentionally or not.

It wasn't the blue chest that had captured my attention, though, as I gathered up Dr. Dee Coulter's neuroscience of music notes. It was the cherry Shaker clock. It was so simple in appearance. A small square clock face floated above the rectangular body. Inside the clear glass door, a plain brass pendulum swung back and forth. It was already ten o'clock, and I could hear Eric and Sebastian putting their water glasses in the dishwasher and getting ready to go upstairs for bed.

"I'll be right behind you," I called as I shut down my computer. "Thanks for starting the dishwasher for me."

"You're welcome," Eric said. "Are you finished?"

"Yup. Done for tonight."

I made one more pass at tidying my workspace. A small loaf

of homemade bread sat wrapped on the blue chest between our pewter wedding candles. A gift from one of my baby moms, I left it for the morning. Beside me was another gift, but from Eric: my beloved quarter-sawn white oak Mission-style sofa table, with all mortise and tenon joinery. Its chamfered table top looked light enough to soar.

The complex-looking table and the deceptively simple clock sat facing each other. The clock was harder to build than the table was, Eric had explained, because the molded bridle joinery in the Shaker clock was almost completely hidden. It was a symphony of subtlety, like Eric himself. Deep things connected beneath the surface calm and simplicity. It was a quality about him I cherished.

Eric was in bed asleep when I finally arrived. I had to turn the laundry over and do a quick once-over on the powder room; one less thing to clean tomorrow before my baby moms arrived for music class. I mopped the floors, just a quick pass. I kept things spotless for them, and I know they appreciated the effort.

When I climbed into bed, Eric had thoughtfully arranged Big Squishy, the Lunk, and the Knee Pillow for me. I made my nest and then I was out. I dreamt of houses. I rarely remembered my dreams, but when I did, I dreamt of houses.

It wasn't always like this. When I was in fifth grade, I dreamed of flying far away. I can still see vivid images of flying over rocky shores. Cool ocean breezes fluttered by my smooth child face and outstretched arms. I felt the rise and fall of elevation as I glided down and skimmed close to the waves, then hugged the air and lifted over the spray-spattered edges between worlds.

I never felt the spray from the foam crashing on the rocks below. Somehow, I knew that it would wake me, the wetness on my cheeks and forehead, and so I flew in soft and cozy breezes. I remembered diving from a height and seeing the expanse of California coastline rushing beneath my slim, weightless body. The shore was always rocky and the sky was always blue.

I can still remember waking from that vivid dream, stunned

and thirsty, on that first morning in the Victorian house in Western Springs. I was in fifth grade. I opened my eyes that first Saturday to a tangle of blue and yellow flowers webbing madly across the ceiling and down all four walls. The oppressive printed strands weighed down like a net cast over the entire space. In the center of the ceiling, a glass orb chandelier, hand-painted in matching blue and yellow flowers, dangled fat and spider-like above me.

My friends called the house "The Mansion of Western Springs," but it was not a mansion. The three-story Victorian was certainly not the largest house in the neighborhood, but it was an impressive home. There were grander homes with wider lots and larger footprints, certainly, but this stately home towered over its next-door neighbors. It was a pillar of classic white with original leaded-glass windows.

Those windows looked out upon a beautiful neighborhood of elegant homes, peacefully intermixed with smaller well-kept cottage types, in a way you rarely find in modern urban planning. Teardowns, they later came to be called. But then, the neighborhood was delightfully eclectic as well as neat and well-kept in appearance. The lawns were green and neatly trimmed and the streets were laid out in a grid, in blocks.

On either side of us, tall elms played London Bridges, forming an autumnal kaleidoscope to filter out the sun. Dutch elm disease was silently striking. I felt as though we had entered an entire alien world, completely different from the dry brown rural hills of California and the sudden flush of orange poppies after rain. The houses were so close together. I missed the smell of pine pitch and meadow grass, and the orchestra of insects in the fields almost immediately after we arrived.

We drove in from O'Hare International in our ugly pea-green Chrysler sedan. Lee Iacocca was in the news with his bailouts. There was a TV sitcom feel to the orderly arrangement of the houses, and the perfection of the landscaping that was so different from the dry and wild fields of Morgan Hill, California. There was one exception to the neatness.

The house three doors down looked abandoned. A haunted place, filled with brambles and bushes that were so overgrown that the house was veiled from sight. Its windows were cataracts, and the paint was peeling off the porch.

Before we were all out of the Big Green Beast on that very first day of our arrival, Isabella Necessary on a Bicycle fluttered in to greet the new neighbors. She was spry and probably eighty, with springy white sprigs escaping from her bun. Her face was friendly in its crinkly bird-like way. Isabella brought us a loaf of homemade bread and told me about her brother, who gave her the nickname years ago and then passed on, I think at the age of eighty-nine. I was simultaneously charmed by her eccentricity and repulsed by her age. I was nine.

Isabella lived for about two more years. After she died, her house was sold, and the new owners cleaned it up and fixed it pretty like the others on the block. But I saw her only on that first day. Though she lived alone and obviously could have used some help, we did not reach out. As Mom often said, she was "not our kind."

The tall white house watched impassively as I talked with Isabella Necessary. The homemade bread smelled yeasty and was still warm in my hands. The large windows observed but did not pass judgment, as though witnessing this ritual greeting, this sharing of food and good wishes. On that October moving day, those leaded-glass windows looked within, too. They cast rainbows across the expensive white silk string wallpaper in the living room and entryway and up over the elegant fireplace mantel. There was a generous entryway with a stately staircase. The banister was beautifully enameled white, with two turns in the ascent.

The previous owners had done much decorating throughout the house, mostly of the very highest quality. The woman actually cried at the closing when they learned that my mom was a smoker.

"My silk wallpaper will be ruined!"

Mom quit that day, cold turkey, and never smoked again.

Neither my older sister's asthma nor the house fire Mom started with her butts at our last house in Morgan Hill were as inspiring as a stranger's disapproval. "What will the neighbors think?" was Mom's bible.

Her oldest daughter's asthma was so severe that she had allergy shots every week in California while we lived there. After one appointment, my sister came home with a new prescription for the asthma. It was a horrible purple concoction. We called it Elix-awful-in, and it was awful. Mom made me take some once when I had a chest cold.

Unfortunately, the medication was not enough to stop my sister's wheezing, so the next step was to lay clear plastic painting tarps all over her bedroom carpet. The doctors said the plastic would protect her lungs from the "dust" in the brand-new shag. Mom taped it all around the edges with duct tape and then cleared the surfaces of her room as well. Knickknacks and collectibles were banished. Cigarette smoke was healthy in the 1970s, but common house dust was forbidden.

One day, while we kids were outside playing in the front yard, Mom came bursting out the front door in a cloud of different smoke. She seized the garden hose and proceeded to put out the kitchen fire herself. Then she called the firefighters, who came out to finish the job. Mom had emptied her gray glass ashtray into the kitchen trash, sure the butts were all extinguished, and then had gone to play piano.

We were all taking piano lessons from the alcoholic neighbor lady there in Morgan Hill. I vividly remember Mrs. Jefferson exhorting me to count out loud, one, two, three, four, as I tried desperately to guess the rhythm of the song.

"What's the matter with you?" she asked in exasperation. "Don't you know the quarter note gets the beat?"

Mrs. Jefferson seemed to think I had another teacher who came before her to do the actual explaining. I remember my second-grade humiliation as I tried to find the answer. *How does a quarter note get "the" beat,* I wondered? I was mystified. *Is it like in "The Farmer in the Dell?" Does the quarter note get the beat like the rat gets the cheese?*

If only she had once explained that the quarter note *equals one* beat, years of confusion could have been avoided and the mathematical logic of musical subdivision could have been implanted in my psyche as a second grader. Instead, I invented my own rhythms, as my quarter notes refused to get the beat like Mrs. Jefferson rejected explanations.

I found Mrs. Jefferson gross and more than frightening. She didn't like me, either. If my rhythm was abysmal, Mrs. Jefferson was a well-pickled metronome. In every lesson, she laid her head in both hands and proceeded to rock back and forth to some internal rhythm that had no relation to my version of "You're a Good Man, Charlie Brown." Sometimes she moaned softly to herself.

Mom decided offering her mints before each lesson was the solution, as she, at least, was learning from this hirsute groaner. Strains of "O Holy Night" were arresting Mom's attention on the day of the great fire. Our lovely Shetland sheepdog, Maggie, was the hero that day. Maggie smelled the smoke and alerted Mom to danger. She barked and barked and led the way, a sable Lassie in miniature.

The actual damage from the fire was small. The trash had caught on fire in the cabinet under the sink, so the flames had burnt an area of probably two feet. The stench of burned linoleum was everywhere, and the smoke damage was extensive throughout the house. The whole house had to be repainted and the carpet all replaced. Mom got a new kitchen out of it, too. Not long after, we moved to Illinois.

So, when we arrived at our Victorian mansion in Western Springs, I think that on some level Mom had learned from her fiery mistake. I want to condemn her for not quitting smoking for our health, but at least she quit. That is something, and while our delicate lungs were permanently scarred, the fragile fabrics were preserved.

It was 1979. I was in fifth grade. There were too many jerks in California, so, like swallows, we had migrated once again. Our limit was usually two, but no more than three years in any one place before the jerks became intolerable. We had been in Darien, Illinois, before the two different houses in California, and of course before Darien was Idaho Falls, Idaho. We kept moving.

In Idaho, I was born, but more importantly, it was where Mom finally had the son she had always wanted. My sister and I both came home from the hospital in blue blankets, swaddled in disappointment. My sister's girlness was less disappointing than mine, though. I think Mom wanted two; a boy and a girl. When my sister arrived first, she was out of order but not unwelcome.

I think I was a burden. My mother had not considered that the unspoken family balance might include an extra female. She wanted one each and that was that. But my unwelcome appearance didn't stop her from trying for a boy, and two and a half years later my brother joined our growing ranks.

The state of Illinois didn't know I had crashed my mother's party, and so it welcomed all of us equally from sunny Morgan Hill with the blizzard of '79 that winter. Jane Byrne was mayor of Chicago and the streets were impassable. I remember walking to Grand Avenue school in the streets, as the sidewalks were buried under glaciers five feet thick.

You would think I would have known what storms awaited when we flew into O'Hare that fall from California. Really, now that I think about it, it's crazy that I wasn't prepared. Children are astonishing in their capacity to forgive, and the protective blanket of denial lays a damp and suffocating woolen fur over things too painful to contemplate. Denial doesn't quite smother the smoldering embers of fear and anger, but rather it banks them in like ancient mastodons buried in the tundra. These dark impulses emerge a millennium later as a clot of tangled emotions, gray and matted, with sharp angry tusks that lurch up out of arctic darkness.

Evil is surprising, too. It lurks quietly, waiting for the moment you least expect it.

Mom had always wanted a Victorian, she told us after she announced the news of the move to Western Springs. She hadn't, of course, but this was her sixth major move in less than fourteen years, all but the first with at least one baby in tow. The role of bride is an easy one, usually. Playing the role of mother is harder. Just ask Medea.

I remember my mom talking about the loneliness and isolation as one of the few non-Mormon mothers in Idaho Falls. I can still hear the wistfulness in her voice as she told me she often sat out on the bench with us and wished that someone would invite her in for coffee.

"But no one ever did," she sighed.

It breaks my heart still. When Sebastian was born, I had a playgroup that met weekly for lunches and outings, Musikgarten classes with friends, mini gym, and park district classes. Eric and I had friends all having kids at the same time. Our children grew up together like cousins. Best of all, we had Marcus and Nancy, who joyfully adopted Sebastian as a bonus grandchild. We are blessed in the love of our friends.

I can mostly see my mom with compassion now. Mostly. She did not drive. After that foot-crushing, bone-breaking, eye-blinding car accident, she refused to drive until I was in third grade, and so not only was she always the new mom on the block, she was literally trapped at home. The isolation must have been extreme.

Mom had three favorite sayings: "Insanity is inherited. You get it from your kids"; "Once is an accident, twice is on purpose"; and "If you don't have anything nice to say, come sit next to me."

Now that I'm a mother myself, I look at my baby book with new eyes, wondering if I was the reason Mom lost her tenuous hold on reality. In my baby book, a yellow, softly padded piece of vinyl, she attached the picture of my arrival at the hospital on the first page. My umbilical cord is clearly there, and she is smiling with her signature modeling eyes, no hint of what was to come.

I am a middle child, so there are a couple of photos actually attached in my baby album and a jumble of photos randomly stuffed inside. I'm not sure, but I think at least fifteen of them are the same professional photo of the ranch house in San Jose, from the realtor.

There is one other photo I recall. It's memorable because it's lovely, but also because it's one of only four of five that are taped in place. It is a picture of a beautiful smiling baby snuggly looking up at the camera from her bouncy seat. She is sunny and an armful of cuddly cuteness; the epitome of the happy, healthy three-month-old.

I remarked to Mom, "Look! I was such a cute baby!"

Mom took one look and snapped, "That's not you, that's your sister."

I think it's obviously me, as I was the one who was born full term, with healthy, non-asthmatic lungs. My sister's face was always thin and sallow; pinched and wary. But who knows? That was the thing with Mom. It was hard to know what was true.

While the pictures in my baby book are mostly a random clutter, surprisingly the childhood milestones are precisely and accurately recorded. Mom kept lists of my words: *mama*, *dada*, *bye-bye*. The list is very long and dated. My verbal skills were obviously significant to her. From the time I was very little, my mother would tell us we were different.

"Genius IQ runs in the family," she said, correctly. "You are smart like us."

The long lists of my first words were proof of my superiority and of her excellence as a mother. I'll admit, we have our gifts. One sibling knits M.C. Escher patterns, and the other sometimes sings professionally. I always did think my gift was music, but now I know it's something else.

My gift is early and extremely vivid memories. I don't mean that I remember the stories of my childhood. Our family rarely spoke of the past. Well, Mom would when she had a grievance; an ax to grind about some imagined slight or unfortunate incident. Nothing bad was ever accidental for Mom. No one ever reminisced about the happy times or the funny stories of vacations gone wrong or the funny time that the dog did that thing.

It shocked me when I married Eric and his family shared

their favorite stories, like the time Eric, three years old, rode his tricycle straight into the pool at their trout fishing resort in Branson. He plunged straight to the bottom, pulled down by the weight of the little trike. His oldest brother David, eighteen or thereabouts, jumped in so quick to pull him out that the money in his wallet didn't even get damp. David tells this story every time we see him, and it's their family history; a verbal marking of their love for one another.

There is only one story from my childhood that I have ever heard.

"You were only a few days old," my mother said, "and I was giving you a bath in the kitchen sink." She paused, remembering the image. "Your sister was two and a half, and she was standing on a chair beside me, singing this little song."

My mom's eyes grew far away as she pictured this cherished scene. She could see it in her mind's eye, and it captured her imagination like a long-lost lover; the one that got away. Dreamily, she told the story, unaware that she was telling me. I would say that she forgot the first rule of theater, know your audience, except that for once she was not acting.

"I was washing the baby and she began to sing this little tune," she said to no one in particular. My mother was no longer present with the current version of myself.

"Wash the baby down the drain."

My mother sang to herself, lost in her reverie. *A little waltz,* I thought, automatically translating the tune to the lilting solfège. *Sol sol mi mi, sol sol mi; a child's tune.*

Then in a child's little voice, Mom said, "Bye-bye, baby!" and she acted it out, waving a precious bye-bye with her fingers curled just so.

The baby she was waving bye-bye to was watching her, alarmed, but she didn't notice. Mom was still singing to herself, eyes vacant. Sol sol mi mi, sol sol mi, and then the darling little wave as she silently mouthed, "Bye-bye. Bye-bye."

It's no wonder my family's stories live more in photos than in words. The less said about the past, the better. I piece together my history from photos and the things I remember. They say the most powerful memories are olfactory ones, and I can attest to that. I have an olfactory memory from my infancy.

My friend and I took our babies to a mommy-and-me baby swim class at the Y. Sebastian was not yet six months old. When I stepped into the cold water for the very first time cradling this precious life to my chest, the smell of chlorine, the cold pool water, and the warmth of his little body clinging to my swimsuit transported me.

For a moment, as I stood with Sebastian in the water, I became the clinger. I was the tiny, fragile body, weightless and cold in the water, my mother's warmth drawing me closer. I remember the feel of her warm skin through her wet swimsuit. I can feel my own tiny fingers clinging to the rolled hem of her scratchy tank-neck swimsuit. Even in this memory, I am afraid she will let go.

Western Springs

I can't let go of memories any more than I can dump a dog on the side of the road. These memories stick, part of the family of my experiences. Like all families, some members bring less joy than others, so I compensate for the unwanted intruders by adopting better friends with whom I build new memories. It's been an extremely successful strategy.

My internal companions, welcome or not, aren't just smells and tactile feelings, or conversations. There's a spatial quality to my early memories as well, an orientation in space, proprioception, too. I feel my location and where things were around me. The first time I walked into my brother's condo in Naperville, I said, "This place has the exact layout of our condo in Idaho, only flipped. The stairs were on the other side." I was right, though we only lived there until I was two and a half. I knew.

Most of my friends don't remember things before the age of four or five, but I do. I retain entire conversations from my toddlerhood, and what's more, I remember understanding the words I was hearing said to me. I also remember knowing what I wanted to say and being unable to form the words in order to reply. I remember the frustration and, unfortunately, I also remember the fear.

I know absolutely that the big vocabulary listed in my baby book is part of it. I remember conversations and events from toddlerhood, things impossible to capture in a photo or a book. Be careful of the words you say, because children do listen, even before they can talk.

I remember lying in my playpen in the condo in Idaho, the one so like its reversed twin in Naperville. The playpen was against the wall in the family room, opposite the stairs. The kitchen was to my left and the front door to my right. I could feel the white nylon mesh of the side of the playpen. I learned to keep my face to the wall and study the patterned quilt below me. It was a cotton patchwork quilt with a puckered edge. It had scenes of kittens playing on it.

I knew that I would be there for a long time, so I waited with eyes closed, deeply breathing. When Mom got up and passed by on her way to the kitchen, I felt her gaze. She stopped and looked down at me. I breathed deeply and exhaled, hoping she would go away.

We left houses, but we didn't leave my mother. I remember each house we lived in. There would be six in all. I was born in Idaho Falls in 1968. The condo there had a pool, where my mother carried me through the water, not yet leaving me to drown.

Two and a half years later, we moved to Darien, Illinois, to a split-level house with yellow shutters and a black-and-white-tile basement floor. I know the floor plan still, though we moved when I had just turned five. Then we moved to San Jose, California, to a large, Spanish-style ranch. Two years later, when I was just starting second grade, we made the hop to Morgan Hill. I was just starting fifth grade when we moved to Western Springs, Illinois. I should have been prepared for what was coming.

We lived out of boxes. Each house got bigger as we moved. The Mansion of Western Springs was just one more size up from the sprawling yellow contemporary in Morgan Hill. Like Mom's outfits, they kept expanding. But the mortgage expanded as well, and no one thought to include the cost of living in Chicago. She lived paranoid and humorless, as well as paycheck to paycheck, and had hardly any furniture to fill the vast emptiness of that white Victorian tower.

I remember those first days of our arrival in Western Springs, like I remember most of my childhood, in vivid detail. Just after we spilled out of the Big Green Beast, the moving van arrived, right on time. I remember my mom's outrage that day. She talked about it for years afterwards. The moving man had tried to cheat her, she insisted that evening over takeout pizza.

"He moaned and groaned as he carried that big box into the house like it weighed a ton, trying to get a bigger sympathy tip!"

Her big eyes flashed tightly, her mouth puckered at the memory of how the moving man had been out to get her. "But I'm not a rube. I saw the writing on the side of the box." She paused, and then put her hands on her hips and barked the answer.

"Lampshades!"

Whether the moving men were cheaters or jokesters, the small amount of California-style modern furniture was quickly unloaded from the moving van and arranged awkwardly in the classic lines of the stately old home. What my mom lacked in humor, she made up in wild decorating. The electric orange and moss-green floral sofas that had looked so dashing against the burnt-umber accent wall in the split-level contemporary in California clashed brilliantly with the cornflower-blue wool carpet in the Victorian living room.

I remember watching my mother direct the moving men to carry the bright orange and green sofas through the wood-paneled family room, which was adjacent to the avocado '70s kitchen, where they would have looked quite nice.

"In the living room," she waved imperiously.

The lead man shrugged at his companion and they carted the furniture into the beautiful cornflower-blue wool-carpeted living room with the white silk string wallpaper.

"Why are you putting those there?" I asked, eyes burning from the clash.

Mom straightened, put her hands on her hips, and snapped at me, "Because they're newer."

She shook her head and turned back to her task, waving in the electric-orange velvet wingback chair to complete the look, as well as the Kimball upright.

"Be careful," Mom told the moving man as she hovered nervously. "It's a good chair. It's from Ethan Allen."

An octagonal game table filled one side of the wood-paneled family room addition. The old comfy family room sofa was slip-covered in a basic navy that didn't go with anything, and a couple of funky orange and plum modern shag rugs that were more than half dog fur created two itchy islands over the smooth hardwood sea.

The family room décor was finished off with an ancient cardboard moving box with a dirty blanket that had never been washed. That was Maggie's bed. The box went at the end of the sofa, tucked behind a brown leather sling chair beside the *Encyclopedia Britannica* collection. A California driftwood clock with brass numerals and a swinging pendulum was later fixed on the wall above the books. Finally, the big wooden TV box with the bunny-ear antenna was placed beneath the pass-through to the kitchen. Channels 2, 5, 7, and 11 were marked with masking tape.

In the eat-in kitchen our modern stainless-steel and maple butcher block dinette set was parked, UFO-like, on a field of olive carpet. Dark-green '70s floral wallpaper covered every wall. Upstairs, the floors had been hastily covered in bright white carpeting before the house had been put on the market. In the 1970s hardwood was a liability and wall-to-wall was all the rage. I got stomach flu shortly after we moved in and puked all over the pristine white hall carpet when I didn't make it to the bathroom in time. The stain never came out.

These are my memories of when we first arrived. I remember it all. I remember feeling nauseated as I sat sobbing at that thick, blond butcher block table. It was Monday. It was my third day living in Western Springs. I should have known better. I should have seen it coming, but I was nine years old and I didn't.

The takeout pizza congealed on my plate as I cried. *I'm a failure. I am stupid*. The sixth-grade crossing guards found me wandering blocks away, completely lost.

"What an idiot. How can you be so stupid?" my mom sneered, eyes like lasers.

"I'm sorry. I didn't know how." *I am useless. No wonder I'm not wanted.*

"That's pathetic."

"How come you don't want me?"

Mom froze, her large blue eyes widened in shock at my temerity. "You are so stupid, no one would want *you*." She drew the vowels out as she sneered, so "you" came out "youuuuuuuwah."

"It makes me feel like I'm not important when you don't come for me on my first day of school." We'd had a family discussion about "I statements" during dinner. My sister learned about them in health class that day, and I applied what I'd just learned.

Mom pulled her considerable bulk backwards, both hands on her thighs. She straightened her back, and with those big blue eyes wide open at my insolence, she said, "You aren't important."

I choked, tears waterfalling down my cheeks, spattering my T-shirt and splashing onto my hands in my lap. "How come I'm not important?"

She jerked back, her head whipping erect and those big blue eyes opened wide. She pulled herself up even taller, staring at me, and then enunciated each word clearly.

"You." Breath. "Just." Breath. "Aren't."

I leapt up from my seat and yanked open the door behind me. As my feet pounded up the servant's stairs, I heard my sister: "Stephanie is so stupid. She is always lost."

Raucous laughter.

***

"Where are you?" Eric called.

"I'm at my desk," I said, as I finished typing my newsletter: "Music forces both halves of the brain to work together through the corpus callosum in a way that no other activity can mimic, which has immense neurological benefits." *Thank you, Dr. Coulter*, I thought.

"I'm going up to bed."

Eric's hands were warm when I reached up, and I leaned back against him.

"Another early meeting?"

"Yup. I'll be out the door by six." His lips brushed my hair.

"I'll be up in just a few minutes. I have to finish my

newsletter." I squeezed his hand, smiled back at him, and turned my attention to my work.

"There are two types of intelligence," I typed, glancing again at my neuroscience of music Musikgarten packet, "fixed and fluid. Schools tend to focus on fixed intelligence, which helps children to understand the facts and figures that are needed to remember the correct answers on standardized tests."

I thought of the enormous number of assessments that Sebastian had dealt with in elementary and middle school that far surpassed what I had experienced as a child growing up. I shook my head and kept typing. "You see fixed intelligence at work when children are asked to parrot answers. Memorization of facts is one important skill," I continued, "but solving problems creatively, especially complex issues that may not have just one answer, requires fluid intelligence."

I explained fluid intelligence, flexible persistence, and how musical improvisation helped children to develop the highest form of thinking skills by allowing them to think creatively, come up with their own ideas, and incorporate them into an existing framework.

I paused and remembered Cathy Mathia's teachings in Dallas and did my best to capture her words as she had explained the neuroscience of music to us. "You are fostering the beginnings of improvisation and imagination," I typed, thinking I had got it right, "all of which take place in the frontal lobes where all higher-order thinking takes place. Imagination is the ability to see the unseen, and the key to all discovery and invention."

I finished the paragraph and turned off the computer. My eye fell on the bouquet of red roses on the kitchen table as I stood. I took a moment to inhale the sweet, spicy fragrance before heading upstairs.

Eric started showering me with roses on our first date, and I handily rejected them. We met on a blind date, back in the day when that was daring. I recognized Eric's kindness in his eyes the first time that I saw him. He brought me a single rose. That's how I spotted him; tall, dark, and handsome in the entryway at

Bennigan's.

He carried that red rose for me, but it was those Duesing eyes that got me. His gaze was gentle on my soul and I think I knew right then that this man was the one. I knew this gentle giant would not hurt me. That knowledge made me nervous. I still remember how anxious I was at that first date. Eric says he didn't get a word in edgewise, I talked that much.

After lunch, as we walked through the parking lot together, I chattered on and on. I couldn't bear that moment at the end of the date when a man used to either say "I'll call you" or nothing. I couldn't take the pressure, so I talked.

"I have Monday off and I'm going to my friend's baby shower tomorrow. I got her the cutest gift! It's a little bear outfit with little ears on the hat. I wanted to wrap it in silver with pink and blue ribbons, but they were all out at Hallmark so I got the green ones instead. What are you doing tomorrow night?"

It was a shocking breach of convention in 1994. Fortunately, Eric rescued me from the awkwardness of asking a man out on a date with a huge smile and said, "Going to the movies with you, I hope." I teased him that he was probably hoping that being in the theater would shut me up. It wasn't until I got home that I realized I forgot the red rose on the table.

I forgot the next one, too. I left it on the floor of the theater the next night, and the next one on a restroom countertop, and one on a restaurant table. I left one in his car. It was like the roses became invisible with this man taking all my attention. Eric came back for me again and again.

I was twenty-two and a brand-new music teacher of uncertain ability and tons of confidence when Eric told me he loved me for the first time. He said something that changed my life forever. He wrapped his long arms around me and looked at me with those perfect Duesing blue eyes, and he said fourteen words: "I want you to know I love you even if I never say it."

He followed that statement with this: "I want you to be able to tell that I love you from the way that I treat you."

One half of me was rejoicing in the present with the man I

loved back. The other half was watching, split screen. In my omnipresent memories, I could see my mother's raging face and hear her shrieking voice: "I said I love you! What *difference* does it make how I treat you?"

A single statement turned me inside out. Eric put into words that day what I had wished for but didn't know existed. He verbalized what I suspected could be possible but had no words to say myself. He spoke love into being through his actions. Eric got a glimpse of my family life at our first Christmas as a couple. He saw firsthand why we kept our family stories buried in the past.

Christmas Gifts

"It just doesn't feel like Christmas," Mom sighed.

I adjusted the phone and sat down on the electric-orange velvet wingback chair, so uncomfortable and ugly that it still looked brand new. Mom had volunteered to host Christmas again this year, and clearly wasn't up for it. I considered what to say.

Nickie jumped into my lap and I brushed my hand over his silky black head. His ears were still puppy soft, and tipped adorably, border collie-style. I ran my hand over his head again, enjoying the silkiness of his bold tuxedo coat; the white fur of his ruff and belly was almost imperceptibly longer than the black plush velour down his back. He whined softly and settled all five pounds of fluff in my lap. His white plume waved gently over my left arm as I ran my hand down his midnight back again.

"I'd be happy to have Christmas at my place if you aren't up for hosting." I tickled the good spot under Nickie's ear. He reached his paw out and hooked my forearm, gentle and catlike. *More petting please*, he said.

"Oh, no. You don't have the space. I always host."

I looked with pride at my large living room. Everything was clean and neat, and my first Christmas tree was sparkling in front of the large picture window. All my ornaments from my first students took pride of place. Two dozen brand-new blown-glass ornaments from the hardware store filled the tree sparsely but cheerfully. I looked at the festive tree with satisfaction and tried for the third time to reason with my mother.

"It's okay if you don't want to, Mom. I am happy to. My apartment is big enough and Eric has a card table. We can seat everyone together."

"No, no," she said breezily. "I want to."

"You don't seem like you are up for it this year, that's all I'm saying."

"I can do this." Her tone sharpened with irritation. "I always host."

My new one-bedroom apartment was a stretch on my first-year teacher's salary, but I had had no choice after the last screaming session when Mom's garbage disposal broke. It was all my fault, she raged, even though I wasn't home when she broke it.

I sheltered for a day or two at Eric's place, and he helped me find the apartment and move in. As I packed to move, Mom became unexpectedly generous and donated the old blue chest, the orange and green floral loveseat and the electric-orange wingback chair.

"Be careful," she warned as Eric lifted it into the U-Haul. "It's a good chair. It's from Ethan Allen."

Once I removed the zippered covers from the floral loveseat cushions and washed them, the gray film of cigarette smoke washed away. With the beige walls and carpet, everything looked nice, if out of date by three decades. *Christmas here would be nice*, I thought, but I knew better than to provoke her.

"Okay, if that's what you would really like. You only have to make the turkey and the stuffing," I reminded her again. "Everyone else will bring the sides and pies."

"I've been thinking of making a sparkling white grape Jell-O salad," she mused, for the fourth time.

I mentally cursed myself for mentioning Eric's mother's creamy gelatin salad at Thanksgiving. I gestured in exasperation at Nickie. He shook his fluffy papillon puppy ears and hair went every which way, giving him a crazy look. I muffled my laugh and he ran his tongue out at me and grinned.

"Mom, you know no one in this family will eat that."

"But it's a really great recipe! You use sparkling grape juice and then the bubbles stay in the Jell-O," she enthused.

I gave up. "If you want Jell-O, then make Jell-O." *Just don't be surprised when no one eats it*, I thought to myself. "Everyone likes our standard Christmas stuff. No one cares that our Christmas dinner is exactly the same as Thanksgiving. We will have tons of food."

I ran my hand down Nickie's back. He asked for more, catlike paw hooked over my arm, pulling.

"Well," she harrumphed, "don't forget the sweet potato casserole. I have to make that for Eric," she said sweetly.

"Mom, I have told you three times already that Eric will not eat sweet potatoes."

"You most certainly did not!" she huffed in her Victorian-spinster-lady-rejecting-an-indecent-proposal voice.

Exhausted, I looked around at my pretty Christmas tree, all festive twinkly lights and the two packs of twelve glittery new ornaments floating amongst the branches. Christmas looked less and less enjoyable every second.

I took a deep breath and exhaled. I rubbed my forehead. Nickie whined and hooked my phone arm. More petting. I changed hands and tried again.

"Yes, Mom, I did. I told you last week and the week before." *And three times already in this conversation,* I thought, impatiently. "Eric does not eat sweet potatoes."

"You said no such thing." This time it was her aggrieved little-girl voice. Pouty.

"Mom, nobody in our family likes sweet potatoes except for us, and I don't need them."

"Eric is from the South," she huffed in her schoolteacher expert voice. "He has to have the sweet potatoes with the marshmallows on top." I could see her nodding a *so there!* through the phone line.

I controlled the irritation in my voice as best I could. "Mom," I said slowly, "we have been over this before. Eric does not like sweet potatoes. He will not eat them."

Nickie leaped off my lap and danced excitedly, then put his puppy nose to the carpet.

"I have to go, Mom. Nickie has to pee."

I grabbed his leash as he squirmed and circled my ankles in a black-and-white blur of fluff.

"You were just out an hour ago," I said, scooping him up and kissing his head.

I snapped his leash on his blue collar and we headed down the three flights of stairs and out, thinking about what Eric had said when I told him I had gotten Nickie.

"A dog will be good practice for having kids."

We walked three miles, and twice, total strangers stopped their cars and waved hundreds of dollars at me, offering to buy Nickie right there.

"He's not for sale, but thank you," I said. "Come on, you cute monster. One of these days you will be potty-trained, and I won't have to walk you every two hours all night long."

***

My mother was not cute on Christmas Eve. Eric and I carted casseroles and dishes to the door and rang the bell. Mom was dripping sweat when she opened the door. Her thick blue terry bathrobe was covered in food stains. The bottom six inches of fabric were gray from dragging across the dirty floors. Her hair hadn't been washed in weeks.

"Are you okay, Mom?" I asked.

"Merry Christmas!" She smiled widely at Eric, then shot a hostile look at me. "Merry Christmas to you, too. It's a lot of work!" She adjusted the robe and tied it tighter around her belly with a hard yank. "This morning I had to decorate the tree, and then wrap the gifts, and then do all the cooking." She looked for sympathy from Eric.

"Merry Christmas, Mom," I said, juggling the Waldorf salad and the homemade cranberry compote. "You left everything for today?" *That's a new one,* I thought, giving Eric an apologetic look over her shoulder.

"Are you criticizing me?" she said archly. "I didn't have any help." She simpered at Eric. "That's okay. Eric understands me, don't you, Eric?" She smiled sweetly at him and then limped back into the kitchen.

Eric lifted his eyebrow at me, and we followed, Eric carrying the fresh green bean casserole.

When we finally sat down at the table, set with Mom's elegant black-and-white china and sterling silver, there it was;

the unloved sweet potato casserole covered in globs of browned and melted mini marshmallows. Right beside it lurked a lump of amphibian Jell-O; hunched and glistening, frog-like, in Mom's best cut-glass bowl. Halved green grapes bulged wart-like beneath the clear wet skin.

"Who wants sweet potatoes?" Mom said in what she imagined was an enticing voice. "I put marshmallows on them just the way you like," she said to Eric, smiling. It was her polite company smile, which never quite met her eyes.

"No, thank you," Eric replied as we exchanged another look across the table. I'd warned him.

"How about some Jell-O?" she tried next, looking all around the table.

There were no takers for that, either. Mom ceremoniously lifted the cut-glass bowl and dissected the Jell-O frog with the sterling silver serving spoon. She plopped a large helping on her plate, where it wobbled flabbily.

We passed the turkey and the sides, made small talk about work and the weather.

"Eric," Mom said, lifting the untouched sweet potato casserole and waving it temptingly. "Are you sure you don't want just a bite? I made it just for you." She smiled her charming company smile.

"No thank you," Eric said graciously. "Everything is delicious. I'm saving room for pie."

Mom's eyes flashed and landed on the cut-glass bowl, which had sat untouched since her surgery. Her smile returned, only bigger. She reached for the bowl of melting greenish slime. Going around the table to her right, she looked at each guest and asked each one individually if they wanted Jell-O. Her tone became sweeter with every rejection, until her smile was saccharine when she turned to me.

She considered me, and then looked at the untouched glob of Jell-O on her plate. She nodded thoughtfully as she put the bowl back down. An idea formed behind her eyes. She picked up her fork, which had been resting in a puddle of gravy, and put it in her mouth, cleaning the gravy off with her lips as she pulled the fork out.

"Mmmmm..." She smacked her lips. "Goody, goody gumdrops!"

She treated everyone to a jolly grin and then scooped a large forkful of Jell-O salad and grinned unpleasantly at me.

"Have a bite."

Gelatin jiggled alarmingly six inches from my face. I shied slightly to the left, trying to avoid the fork and my mother's leer.

I replied politely, "No thanks, Mom. I don't eat Jell-O." I took a bite of dressing, still leaning to the left. "Your dressing is delicious, as always."

She ignored the compliment and smiled harder. She waggled the wiggling mess again in an unappetizing way.

"Just try a bite." Her smile stretched far back, teeth bared.

"No thanks," I repeated. "I have enough."

Everyone's attention was studiously on their plates, except for Eric. He was watching from across the table.

"Just one bite." She fluttered her eyelashes at me flirtatiously. I tried not to notice it in the corner of my eye. "It's delicious."

I turned and looked at her. "I said no thanks."

Her eyes gleamed with excitement. All around the table, napkins were in desperate need of folding, green beans were studiously arranged, mashed potatoes mushed into important artworks. All the conversation died in a desperate attempt to not see what was blooming on my mother's face.

"Just a taste." Her eyes were slits.

"I said no, Mom. Please just stop."

Her eyes lit up and her face danced with something vaguely reminiscent of amusement.

"Have a bite," she insisted, all pretense of hospitality evaporating.

I felt the simultaneous press of cold, wet slime and each individual tine of the fork drilling into my right cheek. The four sharp tines weren't yet punching through my skin, but it wouldn't take much more pressure. With my tongue I could feel four bumps erupting through my cheek into the space between my teeth.

"No," I repeated. I was frozen. *If I try to get up, will she stab me before I can move?* I wondered wildly. I could feel the tines beginning to break the skin. I was trapped with my back to the old sideboard behind me. There was nowhere to go in the small space.

I looked desperately around the table and everyone was arranging silverware, dicing turkey into mincemeat, fussily picking the raisins and the walnuts out of the Waldorf salad. Except for Eric; his eyes were wide, his face alert.

He was about to speak when I felt four sharp points press harder. A glob of gelatin, warmed from my skin, calved from its blob-berg and slid down my cheek in slow motion. It hovered at my jawline, then plopped on the front of my new silk Christmas blouse. The Jell-O gathered there, then slid, leaving a moist trail all the way down. The pressure of the fork did not let up as my mother smiled gleefully.

The glob of gelatin hovered on my chest where it balanced indecisively for a moment before hopping off and landing wetly in my lap. My face was hot. My cheeks burned despite the cold and slimy wetness. I wanted to disappear below the table.

"Just a taste."

She pushed on the fork again a little harder. Her breathing quickened. Her excited eyes dashed across my face. She jabbed again, harder this time.

"Have a bite."

What is the matter with my eyes? I thought furiously. I was burning up and stiff as a corpse. I turned my head and ate the Jell-O off her fork. Her eyes fixed on my face, watching. She exhaled.

She nodded her head firmly with satisfaction and then smiled triumphantly around the not-seeing table. "Who would like some pie?"

Everyone leapt up to clear the table.

Now I'm grateful that Eric witnessed what he saw that day.

"I was just so shocked, I didn't know what to say," he told me later. "I've never seen anything like that in my life. I couldn't get to you from across the table, and I was just about to say something when it was over."

Eric's deeply ingrained politeness from his upbringing kept him from criticizing my mother's behavior in her presence, but I was still overwhelmed that he acknowledged that anything she did was inappropriate. That night was the first time in my life that someone close to me had acknowledged witnessing my abuse. All my life, my mother's deranged behavior was not just excused but dismissed. "That didn't happen," "You deserve it," and my favorite, when absolutely nobody was laughing: "It was just a joke." That one was always followed by "You should be able to take it."

I can't overstate how much it meant to have Eric confirm that, indeed, I was stabbed in the face with a forkful of Jell-O salad at Christmas dinner in front of everyone, and although he was too surprised and shocked to intervene, he didn't lie about it or make excuses for it. At the time, I was humiliated. This madness in my home life was just normal to me. I didn't know anything else. I know now that what we perceive as normal is just what we are used to. Eric showed me a normal that was healthy and loving.

That day that he told me he loved me, standing with his arms around me, I started to awaken. Love is action, not a word. Love is kindness, not a three-word phrase. This basic human truth was new to me. I was blind to the basics of human interaction. I knew how to give love, but I had no expectation that it would or even could be returned.

Everything I had been taught about myself, my unwantedness and worthlessness began to fall away, and I gradually began to see what I had been missing all these years. I had always known my mother was mentally ill, but what I didn't know was the love of a person who was healthy. Eric gave me that; a gift of selfless love.

Eric gave me emotional and financial stability. He was, and

is, a good provider and the center of our household. A software engineer, he made a good living and was truly passionate about what he did. Our bookshelves were filled with thick tomes about software development. His company paid for him to get a Master of Science in computer science.

Eric was smart, hardworking, generous, and kind. Having helped his dad build houses as a teen, there wasn't any chore or project he didn't know how to do. He was handy and handsome as well as very gentle and solicitous of my every need at home.

We both have values, and Eric and I waited for marriage. Eric was raised strict Catholic. At the wedding, one of the guests came running up to me just before we left. Her eyes sparkled maliciously.

"When are you due?" she asked me breathlessly. Her eyes flashed over my stomach in my white silk wedding gown, delighted to have a juicy bit of gossip.

"What?" I asked, hitching my skirts up as I walked over to say hello to the friends at the next table. "What are you talking about?"

"When are you due?" she repeated, assessing my waistline again. I stopped and turned to face her. "I didn't know you were pregnant."

"What on earth are you talking about? I'm not pregnant."

She straightened her back and looked me in the eyes. "Your mom said you're pregnant."

"Are you kidding me?" I looked wildly around for my mother, heat rising in my face. "I'm not pregnant. I have never been pregnant."

This person, who I did not know well, looked at me skeptically.

"She knows that Eric and I are waiting. He is Catholic. Where is she?"

Her face fell. "Oh," she said. "Your mom is out on the dance floor singing 'I'm going to be a grandmother.'"

Sol sol sol mi la sol sol sol mi, my brain translated. I looked up at the dance floor, and there she was, singing loudly, my conservative, faithful Catholic in-laws watching her stiff-faced from feet away. Mom's eyes met mine, daring me to try to stop her. I knew from years of experience that if I gave any sign that her behavior bothered me, she would only escalate her inappropriate behavior. I froze, devastated. Mom smirked triumphantly across the room and then laughed.

Eric saw my mother clearly, while my vision was still blurred. I swam through these silty waters for so long, even my own eyes could not be trusted. People who grow up in healthy families see from healthy eyes. My eyes saw only what they were trained to see: *Everything was my fault. I deserved it. How dare I expect anything else.*

Puppy Love

A child was something I assumed would happen, but I didn't really know how much I wanted kids until we bought a house two years later. I didn't have a life plan worked out, however, when we married, or any timeline. I just assumed kids would happen when we were ready. Honestly, I hadn't really thought much about it at all, in any concrete way, except to know that I was different from my sister because I liked kids.

As a teen, my sister taught me all about Planned Parenthood and the Equal Rights Amendment, and she was vocally opposed to ever having children. I think she had one babysitting job as a teen, and then never did it again. Of course, it was the family who lived around the corner and down the street from our white Victorian. We'll call them the Nowickis.

The Nowickis were a large Catholic family, with four or five active dark-haired kids that I didn't know. I think they went to Catholic school. I'd been babysitting for quite a while before I took that job my sister had rejected.

Mrs. Nowicki was a tall, good-looking brunette. She had seemed slim and fashionable on the rare occasions I had seen her on the street. When I arrived for my first evening with them, Mrs. Nowicki yanked the door open and a cloud of screaming voices came billowing out around her like steam. She was wearing black patent heels, a tidy pair of slacks, and a nursing bra. In her left hand she held her iron, and she jerked it backwards, inviting me in.

I didn't know where to look as she led me into the big house and tried to introduce me to the boil of children. I never learned their names. It was pure chaos, with children flying everywhere and bitter arguments over why they had to have pepperoni on the takeout pizza when everyone knew sausage tasted better. One of them was feeling sick, a wispy little girl in a white flannel nightie, and the rest were a shrieking tea kettle of loud resentments.

Before I could say hello, Mr. Nowicki was vigorously

spanking one of the pizza criers, who only wailed louder. Mr. Nowicki then turned to me like nothing happened and gave me my instructions. The sound of crying rose in the background as though modulating keys. Mrs. Nowicki was at the ironing board, bludgeoning her blouse with fierce percussive strokes. I was trying hard to figure out who was who in all the mayhem.

Moments later, they were out the door, Mrs. Nowicki still buttoning her freshly chastised blouse, leaving me "in charge." The children wouldn't listen, and they didn't like my games. They refused to go to bed on time, and then only in beds that weren't theirs. The wispy one in the white nightgown hugged me tight and said, "I love you." Then she puked at the top of the stairs. I felt a certain kinship.

It would be entirely understandable if the Nowickis were the reason my sister disliked parenthood, except she'd disliked children all her life. She was vocally opposed to reproduction from the time she was a little girl. We'd had the books, Mom saw to that, and many hand-drawn uteruses in ballpoint on a napkin. Mom's wombs themselves had a bovine aspect. Bald-faced uteruses with fallopian tubes arched out to either side like horns blowing ovarian puffs of smoke. Georgia O'Keeffe may have painted reproductive organs as flowers, but my mom made them cattle.

During one such art lesson, Mom told me that when she got her first period, like a 1950s Carrie, she'd thought she was dying or had cancer. I gave her credit for trying to correct this wrong with her own female progeny, though her open-mindedness extended only to the theoretical.

To supplement her bovine wombs, Mom had purchased a book. She called it *The Birds and the Bees*. We kids giggled over the cartoon drawings of the rotund and middle-aged naked couple with their body parts all helpfully labeled, and watched *Free to Be... You and Me*. My sister declared it "gross" and said she would never do it.

She remained adamantly against having children until I was going through infertility treatment, when suddenly she was pregnant. Her baby shower was delightful. I ordered lovely engraved invitations and custom floral centerpieces from Amling's up on Ogden. I got a cake from the Swedish Bakery in Andersonville. It was a beautiful confection of fondant in a white rippled basket weave.

We had a couple dozen ladies of various ages in attendance, and at the shower someone asked my sister if she had tried for very long.

"Nope," she said, "I got pregnant right away."

Mom nodded wisely and announced to everyone, "The women in *our* family don't have problems getting pregnant."

Eric and I did several rounds of intratubal insemination. The doctor told us we had a better chance of winning the lottery than we had of conceiving naturally. One Friday evening I sobbed inconsolably on the couch after one too many unsuccessful tries.

"I don't want to do the treatment anymore."

"Do you want to quit trying?" Eric asked.

"No!" Fresh tears came pouring down.

"Well, those are pretty much the choices," he said, reasonably.

"I know. I just hate it. All of it."

"Those are still the only choices." Eyes gentle, he held my hand and handed me a tissue. I blew my nose.

"I'll call the clinic Monday to schedule the next round," I said.

That next evening, I suspected. I had been wrong so many times before that I told Eric, "I have to run to Walgreens to get a new eyeliner. Need anything?"

Positive.

Eric and I had talked about baby names when we were dating, of course, and we picked out names for the dogs as we acquired them. I don't remember the baby names I liked back then. Teachers find that names get spoiled by their more challenging students. I knew for sure there'd be no Josh, Victor, Jake, or Brandon. Amber was also off the list.

Eric favored Annie for a girl back in those days of theoretical babies, but it had too many connotations of a spunky red-haired waif with creepy empty eyes for me. I still find those original cartoons to be disturbing. Plus, there would be endless questions from new acquaintances: "How cute! Did you name her because of the musical?"

The idea of having a baby was too abstract to contemplate, and so I didn't until we bought our house. We bought an Essex ranch in Woodridge, right off Woodridge Drive. Woodridge is a family neighborhood filled with mature trees and neatly manicured yards. The streets were named after World War II generals: Patton, Arnold, Winston, Dean.

I recognized that Essex ranch when I first saw it. The original peach aluminum siding rose up from the yellow brick all along the front. The Spanish-style entryway was just like the one we had on Lenora Avenue in San Jose when I was five. Two half-brick walls braced the entry sidewalk, with a wrought-iron gate guarding the charming courtyard.

In San Jose, I helped my mother plant baby's tears in the small garden in that little courtyard. Here in the house at Woodridge, there was no room for baby tears. Someone had planted sparkling-white granite pebbles along the walk instead. Later I would place two huge concrete planters on the half-wall, framing the gate. I filled them with coral Dragon Wing begonias to guard our door. I was protective, even in my decorating choices.

Double doors led to a spacious, high-ceilinged entryway that framed a long, comfortable living room that I was never allowed to play in as a child. I knew the orange wingback had lived by the picture window that looked out on the backyard. When Eric and I packed our things to move into our first house, we gave the orange wingback chair and the matching floral loveseat to a neighbor. Although more than thirty years old, the fluorescent velvet chair was in perfect condition. As the neighbors lifted it to take it out the door, I couldn't resist. I locked eyes with Eric.

"Be careful."

Eric smirked at me over the fluorescent fabric armchair and answered right on cue: "It's a good chair. It's from Ethan Allen."

I collected original watercolor paintings from local artists to decorate our new home; the type you buy for $50 and then spend twice as much on framing them. Bouquets and gardens filled my walls, and one line-drawing of an owl. The best part of our Essex ranch in Woodridge was the fenced backyard. It sat upon the ridge of the hill, and the yard sloped steeply down to the houses behind. This house will never flood, Eric and I agreed, laughing.

Although the hill kept water out, nothing could contain Nickie. He grew out of his short puppy coat into a gorgeous, shampoo commercial of a dog. His handsome tuxedo coat grew more spectacularly fluffy, and his big papillon ears exploded comically with every head shake. Nickie was a border collie in a ten-pound package. The book on papillon care, which I should have bought before the dog, stated that some papillons are prone to bizarre attention-getting behavior and could be difficult to house-train.

Nickie was special. I mean that sincerely. He knew the names of every one of his forty-plus toys, without training. He was smarter than us, but he was our special needs dog. We loved him for sixteen and a half years, when I finally had to put him down. I know you'll think I'm cruel when I say this, but even though we loved that dog, it was a relief when he was gone. I'm not a bad person, or a cruel pet owner. I cried at random memories for two years after our pom, Penny, died, so I'm definitely not a monster. Nickie was a challenge.

Nickie could not be housebroken. We tried absolutely everything, both medically and with training, and nothing worked. Fine during the day, this dog required potty trips outside every two hours, all night long, for sixteen and a half years. Eric and I took turns taking him out so that we could each sleep in four-hour shifts. I know it wasn't something that we did wrong, because Penny learned to potty outside within weeks, and Sebastian potty-trained himself at the age of eighteen months.

Thankfully, Penny was perfection in a dog. One single handful of orange sable fluff, she weighed less than a pound of butter when I brought her home. Penny understood the concept of barter. She would bring me Milkbones she'd stashed beneath the couch. She'd stand up on her small back legs, put her paws in my lap, and gently present me with my treat. Then she'd stand beside the door and wait for walkies.

If a dog could have a theme song, Penny's was Wagner's "Ride of the Valkyries." Eric and I would sit in the Adirondack chairs in the back yard and Eric would lob squeaky toys down the steep hill to the fence. Penny would charge down the hill, over and over, and run, full speed back up the hill, triumphant. She was unstoppable. There was nothing we wouldn't do for our sweet Penny.

We called Penny our Million Dollar Dog after she had knee surgery at age two. Six months later, she developed a dry cough and this tough little dog, who wouldn't even cry if you accidently stepped on her toe, cried out in pain if you stroked her head. I took her to the vet five times that week. She had chest X-rays and ultrasounds. By the end of the week, she couldn't stand, and Penny had a spinal tap and myelogram to test for meningitis.

It turned out to be a brain tumor, and they sent her home with us as a quadriplegic. I pictured dragging her around on a skateboard, but we nursed her back to health. Eric expressed her bladder for her because she couldn't even pee, and she learned to walk again a few days later.

We gave her steroids to control the swelling in her brain until she died. The pills kept her comfy but made her ravenous; a fluffy scamper of a shark. She ate her dinner in one bite, then quick as that, ate Nickie's too. He would stand there, looking puzzled.

For Nickie, even filet mignon was examined with a gimlet eye, like a Borgia lapdog examining his water bowl. He was still deciding what, if any, he would taste, when the rabid burst of teeth cleaned his plate in a single swipe. We had to separate them at mealtimes so Nickie wouldn't starve. I'm not sure he cared.

The steroids gave Penny diabetes, but she lived two more years. Eric was an old pro at giving injections after my infertility, so we treated her until the insulin no longer worked. Then I took her in and put her down.

I grieved for Penny like a child. She was that beloved. We called her Penny Loaf, she was such a solid armful of pesky joy. Sebastian was two when she died, and I had Nickie still as well, to blunt the sting of grief. But I know what empty arms feel like, and I know what it means to have a favorite child.

I've read that children know when their parents have a favorite. I knew, and I wonder if Nickie did. He certainly acted like the world was his oyster. He was certain there was a better home for him somewhere else. Any crack in the door was an invitation to disappear. He was off like a rocket and gone until some kind stranger found him.

He was microchipped and had our address and phone number on his tags, because he was lightning fast and adorable to boot. I walked miles calling for him, and I called every shelter in Illinois. I cried so many tears over this dog and somehow, he always came home just as I was thinking about what kind of dog I wanted to replace him with.

Once he was home, he was back to his old tricks. Eric and I joked, "If you love something, let it go. If it comes back, let it go again."

Of course, we never could give up on Nickie, no matter how bad he was. He was our baby. Once I begged the vet for a sedative for Nickie to help him sleep through the night. That night we gave Nickie his medication and went to bed so hopeful that we'd sleep until the alarm went off. But no. Nickie had other plans.

He woke us in his usual pattern, every two hours, to go potty. The only difference was that now he acted like a drunk and tottered sidewise to the door. Like an old man in his cups, he stumbled off the deck and wet himself as he tried to lift his leg and toppled over. Eric and I gave up on medication and just went back to taking turns every two hours, all night long, taking the damn dog out to pee.

As my pregnancy advanced, friends asked, "Are you nervous to have the baby?" "Are you scared to change the diapers?"

Eric and I just looked at each other.

"No."

***

"Bouncing stimulates the frontal cortex of the brain, where all higher-order thinking takes place," I said as I pulled my legs in to sit cross-legged. My arthritis in my right knee screamed, so I quickly straightened it again and sat, one leg bent. I thanked my Musikgarten training and Dr. Dee Coulter mentally again.

Moms and dads bounced and tickled their little ones on their outstretched legs. Laynie laughed, clapping her little hands, and squealed joyfully. Laughter rippled around the room. Jonathan slipped off his mom's knees and toddled smiling to his dad, and then dove in for a hug. Laynie and Harper continued to bounce on their mother Katie's legs. They were bouncing to the beat, though we were no longer singing.

Everyone was grinning at the girls' exuberant joy, so I dropped another one from Dr. Coulter as I pulled the xylophone from its spot beside me.

"Children who are able to keep a steady beat are more likely to be better readers than those who can't," I said casually. All around the circle, parents exchanged reassured looks.

It was time for calming, so I found my starting pitch on the Sonor alto xylophone beside me and began our minor lullaby.

"Bim bam, birri birri bam. Birri birri bim bam, birri birri bam."

My parents knew the haunting minor tune now and joined readily in the singing. I was filled with satisfaction as I assessed my class. I deliberately made no eye contact with parent or child, as to have done so would have drawn unnecessary attention and broken the spell.

Now, after the second repetition, every child was settled and relaxed into the rocking pattern. We singers breathed as one. Out of the corner of my eye I could see Jonathan making the "Buh" sounds in time with his dad. His eyes closed, and the class relaxed into the nothingness/everythingness of the music. Sometimes it took longer, but today everyone was Zen.

"At this time," I said gently, looking down and to the side so that no child felt the pressure of my gaze, "if you would like, you may go behind your grown-up and rock like this." I paused briefly for effect, switching the baby doll that I used as a model from my lap to hang cape-like down my back. I held the baby doll's hands to keep her there, and reassured my littles, "But only if you want to."

I looked down at the xylophone casually as I spoke; no pressure on these tiny humans to perform, and no expectant gaze.

I had my parents trained now to let the littles choose their comfort zone. The adults said nothing and let the children choose how they wanted to rock. Laynie jumped off Katie's knee, looked at Harper, who was already draped around her mom's back, and came to rock on mine. I smiled at her and paused to let her climb on my back for a ride.

The pause in singing was only a moment, and the singing continued almost unbroken. My exhortations via newsletter to take ownership of their own voices as the perfect sound to comfort their own child had fallen on listening ears. My least confident adult was singing to her child. She was in tune with the others. I didn't look at her. I didn't look at anyone directly.

We sang and rocked and rocked and sang. Our voices blended together in a smooth, soft band of hypnotic sound. We were connected to each other, and each parent to their child, in perfect calm. This was love, this was joy, this was hope.

"The children who are sung to in early childhood are the most likely to go on to play an instrument in school," I mentioned as we ended class, remembering my Musikgarten training. "They fall in love with music while they fall in love with you."

I watched, enjoying the final moments with my families. They were all bonded, and the love between them surrounded them both like a halo as one young mom brought her son more snugly into her shoulder and kissed his soft face.

I felt like Mary when Sebastian was born. It was only for a moment, but I remember it vividly. My internal soundtrack plays

"Mary, Did You Know?" whenever I remember these events. What did Mary really know? It's a good question. I ponder these things whenever this lovely melody comes to me.

There in the hospital, with my naked newborn on my stomach, my brain split into two halves. One half, my constant recorder and observer of myself and the events around me, was amused.

You realize you are completely nuts, I remember thinking to myself, as I drank this known/unknown, so familiar baby/stranger in with my eyes. I hadn't touched him yet, and we were looking at each other face-to-face across my stomach.

The other half of my brain was raving: *This is who it is! This is the person! This is the perfect little person who has been inside me.*

I didn't think I'd birthed a god, though, so you can stop worrying about my sanity. You can save that for later. That Sebastian himself could be a miracle never occurred to me as he turned his beautiful little head and looked me in the eyes.

Inaccurate Conception

I knew that Sebastian was only human; a very perfect one, of course, with ten tiny fingers and ten tiny toes. I marveled at him as we stared at each other, as though across a vast distance. Those eyes! Those perfect baby eyes that I had never seen before fixed on mine. *I know you now*, I thought. It was his physical perfection, and the miracle of science, that had my brain spinning.

With my baby lying on my stomach, I felt connected to the ancient past. Generation after generation of cells combining, splitting, growing, for thousands of years. Helixes of DNA, spinning, splitting through the centuries, were reeling through my imagination. I was meeting him for the first time, though I thought I already knew him from his presence in my womb. I felt a connection to the unbroken line of mothers arcing back through the millennia. It was the chain of life that I thought was the miracle.

We see through a glass darkly, but Sebastian was all light. Was Mary ever tempted to brag about her baby, I wonder? I am a proud mom and I am definitely not Mary. I will have to brag about my son to tell my story. I apologize in advance, but if I don't brag you will not see how perfectly he hid himself right before my very eyes.

Sebastian came into this world in a hospital that was under construction, not a small and stony cave. There were drills shrieking through the concrete block in the wall behind my head, not peaceful donkeys or cattle lowing. He was due on September 24, and I had a lunch date with my dear friend Nancy on the twentieth.

"Don't you worry about me," Nancy said the week before, over coffee. "If something happens, you don't even need to call me. Just go straight to the hospital."

Nancy was so proper that she spoke in euphemisms. I looked fondly on her sweet and gentle face. She was always there for me, ever ready with a kind word or a hug. She knew all about my childhood and without hesitation offered to grandparent our child.

Nancy's intelligent eyes, both merry and kind, looked out from beneath her mahogany bangs. She and her "knight in shining armor," as Marcus called himself, held court over the loveliest homemade meals in their beautiful Hinsdale colonial. Nancy loved to cook and fussed over every detail of the presentation while Marcus cracked jokes and set the table.

They were a funny couple. She was tall, like me, and always elegantly dressed in the latest fashions. Marcus was short and funny. While Nancy was modesty and propriety, Marcus was the zinger, always ready with a slightly naughty joke.

"Marcus!" Nancy would cry, scandalized. He would grin, unrepentant.

These two older people discovered each other late in life. A first marriage for both, they suited each other very companionably in their retirement years. Nancy had many nieces and nephews who adored their Uncle Marcus.

"Babies love him," Nancy would say. "They love to grab that big old nose."

She was right. Sebastian loved to grab that big old nose, and Marcus would lie on the floor and play with him. Nancy played piano and I sang, the four of us together after lunch or shopping. Marcus and Nancy knew how to make everyone feel special and adored.

Family is who you choose.

Marcus and Nancy loved to attend concerts and shows. Marcus had been an accountant, and he said that attending the theater gave him something to look forward to during long hours at work. They had season tickets at many local venues. Marcus took Nancy to see *Camelot* for their first date, and so became her Lancelot until the very end.

When Sebastian was just a newborn, they treated us to a performance of *The Secret Garden* at a local community theater. Sebastian slept peacefully through it all in his car seat carrier, quiet and untroubled by the acting. The last show we saw before

Marcus passed was *The Miracle Worker*.

Marcus and Nancy quietly worked miracles in our lives, filling our souls with unconditional love and acceptance. I didn't worry about calling the restaurant to cancel our lunch date after my doctor's appointment, as Nancy had quietly assured me numerous times in her understated way that she understood, "If something happens that day."

Instead, I called Eric, who met me at home. He had arranged the dog sitters and asked the hospital for extra security in case my mother decided to show up. I looked at him with gratitude. *This gentle, kind, and loving man will be an awesome father. I am so lucky,* I thought. We squeezed hands.

The hospital sat grandly behind a row of ancient, gnarled walnut trees. We approached through the back way. The hospital had been under what seemed like continuous construction over the past twenty years, and now the campus sprawled around and between a maze of parking garages.

I had preeclampsia and so I was somewhat anxious when we arrived. Quickly the nurses administered Pitocin to induce labor. Nothing happened for a very long time. When the first pains of labor finally slammed into my back like a pro wrestler, I requested an epidural. The anesthesiologist obliged, but the expected relief never came. I expressed my distress to the nurse, and within minutes they bolused the pain medication. There were a few minutes of relief, followed immediately and urgently by intense nausea.

Suddenly, I was retching, then reeling with dizziness. I heard bells ringing, as though far away, and the anesthesiologist came running into the room.

He leaned down over me and said, "It's okay, close your eyes."

Eric was by my side, reassuring and solid, when I regained consciousness about six hours later. Waking up felt like emerging from yards of soft, warm earth. The first thing I felt was Eric's hand. I was paralyzed from the chest down and couldn't feel the pressure of the nurse's hands as she asked me if I could feel a contraction. There had been no fetal distress, Eric told me, so no need for a C-section. Our baby was okay.

Finally, after hours of feeling nothing at all, I felt him crowning. I told the nurse the baby was coming.

"The doctor will be here to check on you in ten minutes," she said.

"No. The baby is coming now," I said.

Things went swiftly then. The OBGYN miraculously appeared just in time to catch a baby who popped easily into the world after only five or six pushes. Sebastian was unceremoniously dumped on my stomach and my heart went wild with adoration.

Sebastian turned his head and his beautiful blue eyes met mine. Recognition. Nothing can prepare you for the moment you finally meet the person you thought you already knew so well. This person. This incredible, perfect human person was finally here, and I finally knew him. He was covered with birth slime and was beautiful; that face, with the elfin chin and the perfect bone structure.

Like all mothers, I thought I had never seen a more beautiful baby, because he was mine. His head looked perfect, not misshapen, and his little arms and legs were waving. The nurses swooped the baby off to bathe and measure him. Sebastian was slightly jaundiced and needed UV light. He got a nine on his Apgar score, they said.

"That's an A!" crowed Eric.

Eric was tired and disheveled from his night on the recliner and he wept from the combined joy of this new life and the stress of almost losing me. I was cradling my baby and Sebastian was latched on. I was feeling so much like Mary, mother of a miracle, that I was both questioning my sanity and not caring.

I wrapped him in the fringed, pastel plaid blanket from Marcus and Nancy to bring him home. It was snowing on that early autumn afternoon, and bitter cold, and we had dogs instead of wise men. Penny brought a Milkbone and Nickie bowed down in play posture, his magnificent ears his crown and his white plume a robe over his back. They greeted our tiny emperor with gentle reverence.

I sat down on the sofa with Sebastian in my arms. Nickie gracefully appeared beside us and anointed Sebastian's ear with the gentlest of sniffs. Penny swirled enviously around my ankles, too short and chubby to launch herself onto the sofa next to me. She contented herself with putting her paws on my knees and examining the baby, ears cocked and tail wagging. Another Milkbone landed in my lap. Curiosity satisfied, she tucked herself under my feet and went back to sleep.

Those first few days were filled with visitors. It was such a joy to show off our new bundle. Grandma Nancy pronounced Sebastian "a very serious baby." He was. He quietly studied each new person, resting calmly and thoughtfully in each new admirer's arms.

We had lots of practice being sleep deprived, so nothing really changed in that department. Sebastian had his days and nights mixed up and was most awake from ten until midnight. Eric and I took turns bouncing him in the blue IKEA bouncy chair until at last he went to sleep. I sang every song I could think of. Sebastian has been my internal metronome for months now, kicking my bladder along to Billy Joel's "Lullaby" or Chopin's Ètudes on the piano.

In the bustle of adjusting to our new life and all the visits from our friends, I was rocketing between my emotions. I told my therapist I felt like the luckiest person in the world to have this incredible, beautiful baby, but I was overwhelmed by the grief of losing my mother. We talked about how survivors of child abuse love their parents and don't want different parents, they want their own parents to be healthy. Children of rejecting mothers try so hard to earn their mother's love, my therapist explained. I cried every day grieving for the loss of a mother who would never be well.

My mother would never be healthy, my therapist explained. Because she had never met my mother, she could not diagnose her. However, my therapist was able to provide a great deal of insight based on what I experienced. I learned about Munchausen syndrome by proxy and what at the time was called a Type B personality disorder. There are no cures for Type B personality disorders. There are no medications for it, and therapy is ineffective because people with this most severe mental illness are so manipulative.

I agreed. My mother was hospitalized for weeks when I was little for self-injury. She called it her "nervous breakdown." She immediately went off the lithium when she was released.

The isolation of living in remote Morgan Hill made being without transportation impossible, or else she could no longer beg rides to the grocery store from unsuspecting neighbors after what happened when we moved in. My mom took driving lessons and got her license. She was terrified of driving a stick shift, and so the great green Chrysler sedan enveloped her in acres of steel, and also had automatic transmission.

"The medication makes me hazy," Mom said. "I have to stop taking it. I ran a red. I thought of your sister, at home alone." She paused, her eyes far away. "I have a family to take care of. I don't need pills." She looked at me. "I just don't know what's the matter with everyone. Everyone else is crazy."

In therapy I learned about codependency and cognitive behavioral therapy. I learned about scapegoating, a common form of child abuse where one child is singled out for abuse. I learned about family systems theory, too, and how when one piece of the family system goes out of orbit, others often follow. Eric and I did the only safe and rational thing. It was excruciatingly sad, and if we hadn't had his lovely family and Marcus and Nancy's friendship, it would have been unbearable.

It felt as though my mother had died, but she was not actually gone. I simultaneously grieved the death of the mother I wished for but never had, and I celebrated the life of a new baby. Eric and I both were on high alert for danger for those first few days.

The additional security at the hospital had helped to ease my concerns about Sebastian's safety from my mother for those first days, but there was no one home during the day but me once Eric went back to work. I felt flayed and raw. My therapist explained that everyone has fantasies about having the perfect family. Eric and I worked on building family out of safe and healthy friends. We are extremely blessed in that regard. Eric was my eyes during this first year of sorrow/joy.

Daily I checked the street outside for signs of my mother's burgundy Volvo. One day, about two weeks after Sebastian was born, my mom showed up. It was just after Eric went back to work, in fact. I'm sure that wasn't a coincidence. It was always when I let my guard down that she pounced. My mother had an unerring instinct for surprise attacks.

I was cuddling Sebastian on the loveseat in the family room. The doorbell rang, and I stood carefully, mindful of Sebastian's newborn head and neck. With Sebastian cradled on my left shoulder, I rose and walked to the door, wondering idly which neighbor was bringing by a gift or casserole.

I yanked open the heavy door and there she was, looking confused and disheveled, her elegant burgundy Volvo in the driveway behind her. Her top was stained with food and her greasy gray hair hadn't been washed for weeks. There were distinct channels making ridges down each side of her head where the brush bristles left crusted impressions. She had obviously given her slick helmet a cursory whack some time days earlier. The back of her hair was matted and every which way, and it was not better from rubbing up against the Volvo headrest.

For the first time in my life, my mother looked uncertain. The mockery and the sadistic gleam in her eyes were completely missing and in its place was genuine surprise. I had never seen her off balance before. Clearly things weren't going as she had imagined. I was supposed to be begging her for love and begging her to love my child. That's the way her script was written.

She had been practicing her new role of grandmother-to-be with relish. The news of my miraculous pregnancy earlier that year had not improved my mother's mental health. While my friends' mothers guessed what sex their babies would be, my mother wasted no time after my announcement to make predictions of her own.

"Your baby won't be as good as your sister's baby."

I saw something bloom in her eyes at that moment: a realization; a desire; a compulsion; then, a decision. Now, standing at the front door, seeing this grubby ghost vacillating on my doorstep, I was at first stunned into silence. Wordlessly, she seized the screen door with her right hand and swung it open.

"Oh," she breathed, her eyes crawling over Sebastian greedily. "Can I come in?"

The Planets

Mom's eyes locked on Sebastian and she opened the door wider. I gasped, and waves of fear and shock rode up my spine as I stood rooted to the spot, cuddling my newborn on my left shoulder. She shifted her weight and put her right foot in the doorway. Abruptly my paralysis ended, and I grabbed the screen door from her with my right hand and firmly yanked it back towards me, still cautious of my precious baby in my other arm. Mom's foot was wedged stubbornly between the screen door and the frame. We locked eyes, and my grip tightened.

"No!" I said firmly.

I hauled with all my strength on the door, feeling the frame of the screen door bend around the lump of her flat, misshapen foot caught in the middle. My heart raced as I considered the possibility that she would push her way into my home. I yanked harder, mashing her foot between the screen door and the frame. The metal frame whined and popped ominously.

Suddenly, Mom reeled backwards, her one good arm pinwheeling, and she jerked her foot out of the doorway. I slammed the screen door, yanking the handle to make sure it was latched. I turned the flimsy lock hard. We stared at each other wordlessly through the glass. My heart pounded in my chest; both arms now curled protectively around Sebastian's tiny, fragile body. Mom hesitated a moment, shifting her weight.

Oddly, her eyes, those wide-open stretches of blue in every photo, were not surprised. It was as if they looked within herself rather than at her daughter on the other side of the window. Those large and mobile eyes did not see the other, younger mother coiled protectively around her newborn, her new-mother's eyes flashing dangerously and her mouth mashed shut.

My mother's body was statue-still, but her expression moved in a wave beneath the oily surface of her skin. Finally, the troubled waters calmed. She nodded thoughtfully to herself, accepted her new role, and turned away. Her entire body shifted into Poor Carol mode as I watched her shuffle down the sidewalk.

Her shoulders slumped and her head hung in mock sadness; her every movement a simulacrum of dejection as she limped back to her Volvo.

I shut the door and locked the deadbolt. I leaned against the door, shaking and crying. I knew from experience that my mother would treasure this role for the rest of her life. I can still see her, playing her favorite part; her chin tucked down to more effectively bat her lashes at her complicit fans. Her huge blue, oddly tearless eyes are absurdly rounded with mock innocence as she tells her tale, first to her credulous and conveniently distant Canadian family, and then to her small number of friends. It's a stellar performance, and she ends it the same way each time.

"... and she did it for nooooooo reason."

She thrusts out her lower lip in a grotesquely cartoonish imitation of childish sadness while she flutters her lashes, waiting for the standing ovation of sympathetic looks and a big floral bouquet of "You poor thing!" She milked the curtain calls of comforting phone calls and lunch dates for every drop of attention, and then some, for the rest of her life.

Her theatrics were a small price to pay.

Exhaling heavily, I leaned against the door with Sebastian's small body tucked in the hollow of my shoulder. His tiny head rested peacefully by my cheek. He sucked his hand and cooed, and for a long moment I stood there, his fragile weight a blessed burden. I kissed the mist of fuzz on the side of his head, inhaling his sweet fragrance, and I waited for the shaking to stop.

"I will never hurt you," I breathed against Sebastian's translucent mist of hair.

His tiny head and body, so fragile and precious, lay in the nook of my shoulder; so perfectly fitted. He was the piece of me I didn't know was missing until he was there, perfect and whole. The enormity of my mother's illness filled me as I hugged his cherished weight against me. I wrapped my hands around him.

"I will never let her touch you. I will never, ever abandon you."

I pulled myself up away from the door and stood up straight. I kissed my son and held him close. I had set a boundary with a woman who had none. My baby's life depended on it.

***

Katie laughed, sweeping Harper into a hug. The mother and baby looked into each other's eyes joyfully. Katie could probably teach this class, I realized for the hundredth time. She was so playful and loving in her musical interactions with both girls. Harper pulled out of the hug and continued bouncing to the beat on her mom's outstretched legs. Big sister Laynie smiled up at me from her place on my lap. I gave her a quick hug too, enjoying the moment with this very musical little person.

"Children who engage in music in early childhood have better balance, coordination, and proprioception than children who do not," I reminded my toddler class parents as I flipped to the next page in my small ring binder songbook. I mentally thanked Cathy Mathia and my Musikgarten training in Dallas and Chicago.

"Another song!" Laynie clapped her hands and bounced on my legs. She smiled up at me and I grinned back, our eyes conspiratorial. *Another song, indeed. At your service, precious one.* I gave the parents one more tidbit while the rest of the class settled.

"All those things help children to succeed athletically." I tapped the mallet on my xylophone, checking my pitch. Still in tune. I sang softly: "My Bonnie lies over the ocean."

On the second word, all the adults, plus Laynie and little Marshawn, were singing this familiar folk song with me. Laynie leaned back against me. I circled her waist with my arm for support and we rocked gently side to side. Katie and I exchanged a look. Katie was grateful for the help and I was grateful for the baby fix with this amazing child. I loved having a teen, but they don't usually let you sing and rock them in your lap.

The fathers' deeper voices added a rich dimension an octave

or two lower. The toddlers snuggled into their parents, or smiled, or looked with interest around the room.

We sang two verses seated. When the melody and tempo were well established, I invited everyone to stand. Laynie jumped up immediately from my lap and held her arms out to me. I lifted her onto my hip. We stood and rocked from side to side for a verse, then I tilted her across my forearm and gently flew her into the center of the circle and then back.

Laynie sang, in tune with the adults, "Bring back! Bring back! Oh, bring back my Bonnie to me, to me!"

The parents swiftly copied my shift in movement, excited for this favorite activity. Babies and toddlers gently and safely flew towards each other and then back on the macro beat of this rocking compound meter. They made eye contact with each other in delight as they swung into the center of the circle. Katie and I partnered up, swinging Laynie and Harper towards each other. The sisters made eye contact and laughed with delight.

The parents enjoyed the reaction of the children, and soon everyone was partnered up; babies and toddlers swinging up to other small children and parents singing and enjoying.

My arms were tiring after two verses of the flying workout. I brought Laynie back to my chest and switched to rocking side by side. She snuggled into my chest and shoulder. We rocked simply, calmly, for a verse or two. Time to calm, time to reconnect, to re-center. When we sat down again, Marshawn signed "more" to his daddy.

As I put the classroom percussion instruments away after class, I remembered Sebastian sitting in his booster seat by the patio doors. It was May 2004, and he was feeding his breakfast to the dogs. Nickie wisped between the legs of his chair with his white plume arched tightly over his back while Penny raced in circles around it, yapping.

Sebastian laughed and threw Cheerios on the floor. One landed in front of Nickie. He froze, stiff legged, and sniffed it like it was a bomb about to go off. I honestly didn't know how he survived in this household. Nickie was made of fur and urine.

Penny almost knocked him over in her rush to get the snack, and Sebastian laughed with delight. Nickie circled back around, wondering when the edible food would be coming.

"Ninny!" Sebastian cried happily, enthusiastically slapping the top of his head with both banana-smeared hands. "Keggy!" He giggled, bumping each pointer finger against his temples.

Oh, do I regret making up those signs for the dogs' names, I thought. *I will be washing food out of Sebastian's hair after every meal for the foreseeable future.* I sighed, and then laughed at his joy and Nickie's confusion.

"Are you all done?" I asked out loud, signing "all done" at the end.

Sebastian picked up one more Cheerio with his precision pincer grasp and ate it happily. "All done!" he signed emphatically, then reached his plump hands to me to get them wiped.

I lifted the plastic placemat with the remains of his breakfast away and then wiped his face and hair with the washcloth. He smiled happily at me as I wiped each little hand. Sebastian's bib kept the worst of the mess off the front of his red shirt, but his sleeves were soggy.

I grinned at him as I unbuckled him, and then I stripped his top off. His little shoulders were muscular, and I swooped his long, slender little body into a hug. A shower of Cheerios hidden in the folds of his pants rained down, and Penny exploded into a feeding frenzy. Nickie tried to tackle Penny from behind for a surprise attack, growling ferociously while mouthing her ears like an octogenarian would a ripe banana.

There was never any bite to his bark, but there was banana on Sebastian's pants. I stripped those off as well and gave him another, longer hug. My shirt was already stained, so why not? I drank him in and kissed his soft cheek. I smelled his sweet toddler smell, now perfumed with banana and the weird, faintly burned smell of Cheerios. Sebastian wiggled for down, and I released him gently, reluctantly.

Sebastian stood shirtless on the kitchen floor. The light from the patio doors made his fuzz of blond a bright halo, and his short bangs wisped appealingly around his expectant face as he pointed to his easel.

"Do you want to paint?"

He smiled up at me and clapped his hands, then hugged himself in anticipation. I settled the paint cups into the Playskool easel tray and attached a sheet of paper. Those beautiful little hands reached up and grasped the chubby paint brush. While I washed his plastic placemat, he made brilliant blots of color. I smiled at Sebastian.

"Bird," he signed, making the beak motion with his fingers.

"Yes, that does look like a bird!" I agreed, signing "bird" back to him as I said the word.

Quickly I slipped the paper out of the clip before he could ruin it and set it on the brown oak dining table to dry. I wrote, "Sebastian's first bird."

I clipped another piece of paper to the easel, and he started another picture. I got one more bird before he lost interest and started painting on himself. He made blue swirls across his tummy and a bright red stripe up each arm. We were going to have to finish painting in the bathtub.

Bathtub painting was much more satisfying for Sebastian. He spent hours every day in the tub. We finger painted and used bathtub crayons. Once when he was very small he swept blue paint over each shoulder and said, "I am putting my overalls on."

He was speaking in full sentences when he was not yet two, but he would continue to use sign language well into second grade. He would be the one on the first-grade soccer team turning cartwheels and picking dandelions. When I'd ask if he had fun at the match, he would be enthusiastic.

"Yes, Mom! I'm making sign language for fairies."

Other children will scrum around him vying for the soccer ball like Penny after a Cheerio. Sebastian will run in circles and bring me a bouquet. Out of desperation, I will promise him a Beanie Baby if he makes a goal. I'm an awesome mom that way. Five minutes later he will be chugging down the field and sinking his shot. Then he will want to know if he would get a toy for every goal, of course.

But I didn't know any of this yet as I was sitting in the exam room with Sebastian waiting for his two-year check-up. Sebastian whirled his blankie around like a windmill and ran happily around the exam room.

"Doctor Fredericks, Doctor Fredericks!" he chanted, like he was rooting for the home team.

"Why don't you come up and sit in my lap?" I caught him around his middle as he dashed by and swung him giggling into my lap. I planted a kiss on his cheek and then blew him a gentle raspberry on his neck. He giggled and twisted away, sliding down my legs, and turned to face me.

Dr. Fredericks was our family doctor and I smiled to myself, remembering how she had spent more time with me on the phone on a Sunday morning than my OB did in those first few weeks after I had Sebastian. I cried on the phone to her and told her my armpits felt like hot pokers were jabbing them after every feeding session. Sebastian had thrush, mystery solved.

The exam room door opened, and a medium-sized natural beauty poked her head in.

"Hello! What brings you two in today?" Dr. Fredericks's lip-balmed smile revealed perfect white teeth. Her shoulder length, curly hair was pulled back in a neat ponytail. Her naturally glowing, liberally freckled skin was radiant without a hint of cosmetics.

"Just a two-year wellness visit."

Sebastian dropped his board book on the floor, slid off my lap, and ran to Dr. Fredericks.

"I know all the planets!" Sebastian boasted.

"Really?" Dr. Fredericks's farsighted green eyes looked even more comically large behind her gold framed lenses.

"Mercury, Venus, Earth, Mars, Jupiter, Saturn, Uranus, Neptune, Pluto, and UB 313!" Sebastian raised both hands over his head and grinned triumphantly. He clapped his hands and said, "You can see them with a telescope. We went to the Adler

Planetarium."

"You did? What does the telescope do?" Dr. Fredericks asked, eyebrow cocked.

"It makes things that are far, far away look closer."

"That's right. How does it do that?"

Stumped, Sebastian chewed his lip.

"It has a lens, like your eye." Dr. Fredericks explained kindly.

Sebastian pointed at his eyes, then sang, "Head, shoulders knees and toes, knees and toes," touching all his body parts.

Dr. Fredericks laughed. "That's right. I'm going to look at your eyes with my light right now. Is that okay?"

Sebastian wiggled and kicked his feet against the exam table. He looked curiously at the light. "Okay."

Before the appointment was through, Dr. Fredericks sketched a careful drawing of an eyeball for Sebastian. He watched in fascination as she drew a medical profile, with the iris and pupil, then showed him the lens. She finished with a little stick figure of a man and flipped the man upside down on the back of the eye.

"More!" Sebastian signed, when Dr. Fredericks finished.

"Is he deaf?"

I laughed, sweeping Sebastian into my lap and giving him a quick hug and kiss. "Oh, no!" I quickly reassured Dr. Fredericks. She relaxed, and Sebastian squirmed in my lap, so I let him down again. "You would have noticed if he was," I joked. "We just do sign for fun."

"Why sign with a hearing child?"

I explained to Dr. Fredericks about seeing a presentation at a mom's group at the local hospital on signing with babies. It was 2001, before signing with hearing babies had really caught on. I was an early adopter. I thought about my early memories, and the frustration I felt as a toddler when I couldn't say the things I needed to express. I didn't share those thoughts.

Instead, I said, "They used to think that signing with a hearing child would impede their language development," I told her. "But it turns out it's the opposite. They learn to speak sooner and have a bigger vocabulary. Signing creates dual pathways in the brain. It creates more neurological connections."

Sebastian had so many words at the age of two, and more every day. He was so verbal. I thought about recording all his spoken words and signs in his baby book, but somehow I just couldn't. I thought about writing them all down, but when I pictured my own yellow, padded baby book, with all the photos of that house in San Jose and so few of me, and the long, long lists of my own words, carefully recorded, I couldn't. My words were my mom's accomplishments.

I heard my mom whispering, "Genius IQ runs in the family, and you are special too. We are different from other people."

Reading the Signs

Sebastian wrote, and early. Not only was language exploding all around us, but also our stuff. You could say the writing was on the wall for a while. Our three-bedroom Essex ranch had no attic and no basement. We were out of closet space.

Eric and I made a deal when we first got married. I wanted to be a stay-at-home mom. Teaching is a much more demanding career than many people realize, and music teachers work long and often unpaid evenings and weekends. Festivals and concerts, contests, musical rehearsals and performances; they all leave little time for family life.

Eric worked long hours, and it seemed financially better for one of us to just stay home rather than pay for daycare. I earned less, and I wanted to enjoy my time with my baby after years of infertility. Eric was one hundred percent supportive of that plan, and he worked incredibly hard to make it possible.

Just after Sebastian turned two, we made the jump to a two-story colonial. It had a half basement with space for Eric's woodshop, and the area's schools were well-known for their music programs. It was still a modest house, a four bedroom instead of three, but it had more square footage.

Our new home had a tiny kitchen but made up for that flaw with a two-story deck that we joked was large enough to view from space. We named it Moby Deck and planned lots of summer parties. The neighbor two blocks down made the same observation at every party: "Your husband has a really big deck."

Eric began his second master's degree program and two years later earned his MBA. His effort made our lives not only possible but so enjoyable, with plenty of fun activities, meals out, and every class or sport Sebastian or I wanted. Eric indulged us, and I was grateful and felt very blessed to be able to spend time with my only child.

Soon after our move, Sebastian started expressing anxiety about going places, like the grocery store and gymnastics class. He called it the "I'm Nervous Game." He would say, "I'm nervous" over and over as we drove to the store or gymnastics class. When I asked him why, he said, "I don't know, I'm just nervous."

I talked about it with Dr. Fredericks at one appointment. She said it sounded like an unhealthy game and that sometimes toddlers can get fixated on an idea when it brings them negative attention. She told me not to encourage the behavior and to try distraction with something else.

Dr. Fredericks was right. Not feeding into Sebastian's anxiety worked, and Sebastian's "I'm Nervous Game" stopped. *Now, if only we can get Sebastian to sleep in a little later*, I thought. Every morning at 4:45 a.m. he woke me, his little face peeking up at me from the side of the bed. "Mommy, I'm ready to play with you."

God bless all parents of these early, early risers. Sebastian and I had five hours a day of one-on-one quality time every morning. I had to get creative with our games. We played outside on the jungle gym Eric and I built in the backyard, and we went to parks. We read, we did crafts, we did more crafts.

When craft time was over, we did painting and drawing, and then there was sewing. Let me be clear. I don't sew. Sebastian asked for a sewing machine for Christmas when he was two, and Eric got him one. I thought about fleeing the country. Many hours were spent playing quietly together in the family room or down in the basement.

Once, Sebastian pulled out a dozen or so of his favorite plush animals and set them in a ring around us. "Let's play school," he commanded, my darling little dictator.

"Okay, teacher."

I picked up his Magna Doodle and drew the outline of a capital letter "A" in dots. I showed Sebastian how to connect the dots into the letter, and then let him do it himself. We did each capital letter once, dot-to-dot. A few weeks later, Sebastian asked to play school again. We read stories and then he grabbed the Magna Doodle. "Do the letters again," he commanded.

Obediently, I drew the dots and he connected them; each capital letter once. Two weeks later I took him to play at the local playground just a few blocks from our house. It had an unusual slide with large rollers, like an assembly line might have, and we laughed at the rumbly vibrations as we slid down together.

"Again, Mama! Again!"

We played outdoors all morning on that sweet spring day. Sebastian was two and a half years old. On our way home we walked through the sand volleyball courts. Sebastian picked up a stick and began writing.

"A," he said, and drew a perfect capital A in the leaf-strewn sand.

"B," he said. He drew a capital B.

"C." Then "D. E. F. G. H. I. J," he continued, writing each capital letter perfectly in the sand. It was not until he got to R or S that he started to make things up.

The early spring sun felt sharp on my winter-pale face as I stood behind Sebastian and watched. I felt the skin on the back of my neck prickle. It was like the sun shining in from the kitchen window at the ranch on Lenora Avenue in San Jose. I remembered sitting at the kitchen table eating breakfast with the blue-and-white half-gallon milk carton in front of me.

I was five and I knew all my letters individually, but I couldn't see the "MILK" on the carton. Mom said it was there, but I couldn't see it. The white half-gallon milk carton had bright blue lettering on the side. I could see all five letters, one at a time as Mom pointed to each one and traced them. First the "M," then the "I," but when I tried to see the "MILK," everything disappeared into a random pattern.

Instead of a word, I saw the white negative space between a bright blue geometric pattern of the letters, like an Aegean Greek key design. I remember the moment the blue letters came to the forefront of my attention. It was as though the blue-and-white design melted and reassembled into meaning. One moment my eye perceived the white background as the focus; a lovely pattern, nothing more. Then it changed.

My focus changed, and in that one moment, a meaningless jumble of color and space became a word. I read at the age of five.

Sebastian was two and a half. I knew at that moment Sebastian had abilities beyond my own, but it would be almost twelve and a half more years before I would truly read him.

By the time he was four, Sebastian was reading and understanding the original Nancy Drew series that I remember struggling with in second and third grade. But as a two-year-old, he was teaching himself, without instruction. There were no drills, no worksheets, no practice booklets.

At the age of two and a half, Sebastian was a furnace of desire to understand things. He was absolutely fascinated by the solar system and we couldn't check out enough books at the library about it. We drew it and painted it and built it out of Styrofoam balls. We made the sun and planets out of papier-mâché and painted them.

Sebastian's thirst for knowledge was not limited to outer space. He loved everything about being here on earth as well. By turns, we went through trains, dinosaurs, butterflies, spiders, and birds. His fascination with nature was constant. He loved to help me in the garden. As I turned the earth over, Sebastian found the worms and put them all into a hole we had dug together.

"What are you doing?" I asked him, as he laid the seventh worm down gently.

Sebastian was muddy up to the elbows, and the seat of his blue shorts was caked in dirt. He turned his bright eyes to me briefly, and then spied another worm wriggling in the fresh turned earth. He plucked it carefully out of the ground, stretching it gently as it came, and placed it lovingly in the palm of his hand. The worm searched eagerly for a place to hide as Sebastian examined it carefully.

Then he delicately picked up the unhappy worm between his thumb and forefinger and carefully placed it in the hole with its cousins. *This kid will have an awesome immune system,* I thought for the thousandth time.

"I'm making a playdate for the worms," he announced.

***

I didn't have playdates growing up. Our gypsy life very purposefully kept anyone from ever getting close to me, and I learned the enormity of the earth and heavens as a six-year-old when we moved to Morgan Hill. The jerks were encroaching again, and so it was time to move from our comfortable ranch house on Lenora Drive in San Jose.

Our next-door neighbors in San Jose managed to produce two completely opposite teenagers. The daughter was a gorgeous slip of a girl. I adored her on the rare times she babysat. Her brother was headed for jail, or that's what Mom said. Mom said she saw the teenage son peeing through the open driver's-side window on to the front seat of our parked car. That was the end of living in San Jose.

"Too many jerks."

I was six and had just started second grade. In a couple of months the house in San Jose was sold and all our belongings were boxed and loaded into a rented trailer. Mom hovered anxiously as the orange wingback was wrangled into place.

Our neighborhood in San Jose had been a typical suburb: house next to house and green lawns. Morgan Hill, although not far from San Jose, was all wild meadows and forest on a high hill. A few brand-new houses stuck up here and there, far apart from each other and set back far from the road. Some houses stood open to the wind, clear plastic sheets blowing around the timber frames like sheets on a cheap Halloween skeleton. The blue eye of the reservoir blinked in and out as we drove past fringes of pine.

"There's our house!" Mom pointed a finger towards a yellow house with dark brown trim far down the Lake Anderson side of Morgan Hill. "It's a California contemporary. I've always wanted a contemporary-style house. It's so modern."

Waking up in Morgan Hill was me in my twin bed, scratchy new sheets, and sticky gray pine pitch still on my hands from climbing the tall pines out back. I ran my hand over my new

Marimekko bed set, feeling the catch of the fuzz of fabric on my sticky palm. My comforter was yellow, with huge orange and yellow butterflies with black bodies. My new scratchy sheets matched the comforter. The best part of all was the royal-blue velvet upholstered headboard. It came from a garage sale, but it was all new to me and silky soft where my hand touched it. It was called tufted, because of the buttons.

Breakfast was grouchy Mom and Kellogg's Raisin Bran.

"Where is everyone?"

"Your brother started preschool. The neighbor down the street is driving him. Your sister goes to a different school. Kindergartners, first and second graders go to your school, and the third through sixth graders go to a different building." She slammed the milk back in the fridge. "Your sister left an hour ago."

"Oh." I ate my cereal quietly.

"Put on your shoes. It's time to go." Mom snatched my bowl away, sloshing milk on the table. "Ugh. What a mess. And the phone installer man isn't coming until tomorrow. That's all I need. One more thing. You're going to be late. Hurry up."

Tall, fragrant grasses as high as my waist lined either side of the road as far as I could see as we walked to the bus stop. Lakeview Drive curved upwards, a black stripe on the back of a winter-coat donkey. There were no sidewalks. I felt the gravel of the shoulder of the road through the thin soles of my worn-out Mary Janes. I walked on the edge of the road behind Mom up the neck of the donkey towards the head. A tall pine in the distance poked up like one single ear on the left.

Mom breathed hard and limped as she walked. A cow in the pasture across the street looked at us as we passed. It was a long walk up the hill. I smelled the bus stop before I could see it.

"Someone is smoking a pipe," Mom said.

The pipe smoke was sweet warm candy in my nose. The cold morning air sent shivers up my back, and I pulled my windbreaker zipper up higher. When we finally got to the top of the hill, in the distance I could see the bus stop. The bus stop was at the base of the tall pine tree, with a small group of people waiting all around it. A big brown-bearded man stood, curls of white pipe smoke wisping softly in the chilly air, and a few grown-ups and active big red-haired boys stood around laughing and talking.

Mom stopped at the top of the hill to catch her breath and didn't go closer. I looked behind me for our yellow house with brown trim, but it was hidden in the deep valley, out of view. My stomach hurt. "I'm scared. I don't want to ride the bus."

Mom whipped her eyes at me and turned her large body between the families in the distance and me. I could not see them, and I knew that they couldn't see me. "You have to ride the bus."

"I'm scared."

"Don't be a crybaby."

"I'm not crying." A tear slipped out. Immediately, her fist came down on the top of my head.

"Stop crying." She glanced behind her furtively to check that no one saw. She turned back, her eyes hard. "You are embarrassing me!"

I rubbed my eyes furiously. Tears were bad. I was not allowed to cry. I was bad. *I was a bad little girl,* I thought furiously to myself. I forced my lips into a smile as more tears dripped down my cheeks.

"Look, I'm smiling." I said between gritted teeth, my cheeks hard and pushed upwards to my leaky eyes.

I heard the bus coming. The engine was loud, and it squealed as it hissed to a stop. The bad smell of exhaust mixed with the sweet pipe smoke. I heard happy goodbyes, and someone shouted, "See you later, alligator!"

"In a while, crocodile!"

"Will you come back to the bus stop to meet me?" I asked. Mom looked at the bus and then at me but didn't answer. "How will I know how to get home?"

Once Is an Accident, Twice Is on Purpose

I kept my cheeks pushed up hard to my eyes, my lips stretched wide, and waited for an answer. The chill breeze dried my teeth and my cheeks. Mom thought for a moment and then glanced behind her. With her left arm straight down at her side, Mom shielded her pointer finger with her large belly. Twisting slightly to the right she pointed with the hidden finger.

"Just follow that kid in the jean jacket," she said.

I got just a glimpse of a red-haired big kid as he disappeared into the bus. More kids piled in behind him. Still with her back to the bus stop, Mom grabbed the front of my jacket. "You come straight home. Do you understand me?"

My eyes widened. Where else would I go? I didn't know a single soul there. I tried to breathe and couldn't. She tightened her grip and leaned down closer to my face.

"You come straight home. Do you hear me?" She shook me a little with each word. "You don't talk to anyone and you don't go anywhere else. You come straight home." She repeated the words. *Straight. Home.* She scooped her chin with each word, making each sound like a bullfrog.

I couldn't find my breath. Her eyes were hard on my eyes. I nodded, nodded, trying to pedal backwards away from her but imprisoned by her grip on the front of my windbreaker. Yes, yes, I nodded. I will come straight home. I will not talk to anyone. Quick as a snake she popped me hard on the top of the head with her other fist, her big body shielding her actions from the small assembly in the distance behind her.

Behind her, the last kid climbed onto the bus. My mother quickly bent down and hugged me to her, licking her lips all around with her pink tongue. She pushed her slobbery wet lips out big and planted a dripping wet smack on my cheek, still holding my windbreaker.

"Ahh!" I wiped my face, hand wet with spit, and rubbed the

slobber in a long, dark trail down my pant leg.

Mom smiled, eyes dancing weirdly, and laughed, but didn't let go. She smiled a big toothy smile and turned towards the bus. She released her grip on my jacket and pushed me between the shoulder blades, smiling bigger as she turned for the dwindling audience behind her.

"Have a great day, sweetie!" She waved a big friendly wave.

I stumbled from the push and then ran towards the school bus. The small group of adults had dispersed, and I was the last one to climb up the big steps. The plastic tang of vinyl seats filled my head as I flung myself to the seat right behind the bus driver. I wiped my face again and scrubbed my hand against my thigh. A brown-haired boy popped his head over the seat.

"It's the new kid!" he called. "Yup! She's crying! Crybaby!"

***

"How could a big girl like you sit and cry at your desk that way? For shame." Mrs. Boda was old, with white hair, wrinkles, and a bun. I stopped crying.

After school, I tied the sleeves of my windbreaker around my waist and then Mrs. Boda took me with the rest of the second graders to the bus line to get on the right bus. I rode alone in the front seat with my Scooby-Doo lunch box, away from the shouting, rowdy big kids in the back. It was a long ride home across a long flat highway, and then the back-and-forth climb up Morgan Hill. Twice, the bus driver stopped on the side of the road, stood up, and yelled. "You kids be quiet!"

At every stop I looked up at the passing stream of backpacks and instrument cases that flew over my face for a boy in a denim jacket, but it was California in October and it was warm. No one was wearing jackets in the afternoon. I looked out the window and searched for the big pine tree by my stop, but the pine trees grew all over. I could see out the door of the bus at each stop, and Mom wasn't at the first stop, or the second. She was not at the third one, either, or the fourth. I was bad, because I wanted to cry.

At the last stop, there was only me and one other little girl. The skin on my face carved itself into stillness. I was not allowed to talk to anyone, and I had to go straight home. I was afraid of the mean bus driver who yelled constantly. He was a stranger.

I was not allowed to talk to strangers. Little girls don't talk to strange men, that was the rule. When the other girl got off, I followed her, my movements stiff and hard. I would not cry. Crying was not allowed.

The bus pulled away in a roar of stinky smoke and faded into the distance, and I was a wooden child. There was no traffic. I could hear the insects singing loudly in the long pasture grass that lined the road. The cow pasture was on my right, but I couldn't see a cow with my hard wooden eyes.

The afternoon sun was shining, and the golden grass waved in ripples with the light breeze. The air was fresh and smelled sweet and herbal. The donkey's back stripe of road was way up high. I shuffled my feet and looked down at the gravel on the shoulder of the road. I kicked a pebble and it bounced off the shoulder and disappeared into the tall grass on the side.

The brown-haired girl invited me to play at her house. I told her that I had to go straight home.

"Are you crying?" she asked.

"No! I just don't know how to get home, that's all." I wiped my face.

She told me I could call my mom from her house, but the phone guy wasn't coming until tomorrow, and I was afraid to break the rules. I said no, again. Going straight home was the rule.

"Well, this is my house." The girl looked at me for a moment, and then shrugged and turned into her driveway. "Bye."

My cheeks were wet. *I am not crying*, I told myself. *I will not cry*. I brushed my face angrily and looked for Lake Anderson on the other side of the road. It was hidden by trees. I could see down the slope of the cow pasture to my right, far across the flat fields way below towards where my school was, somewhere very far away. I could hear the faint sound of the Emerald Regime marching band from very far away, floating up the side of the hill from way below.

In the distance there was a new house up ahead, beams open to the air. Tatters of clear plastic flapped in the slight breeze. Deserted, the empty shell was just bones, like ribs. To my left the ground swept down steeply. The insects sang circular descending cries so loudly, and the grass smelled sweet when I brushed the long stems with my hand. I put one foot in front of the next and kept walking. I had to go straight home, and I didn't know where home was.

My head felt like a pincushion with a million long pins jutting up in all directions. If I reached my hand up and touched my hair, I thought I would feel it standing straight up, ten inches from my head. It felt that tall.

All around me I could feel the whole of the world extending in every direction. I was tiny, an ant, a speck, and nothing was holding me to the surface of the earth. The world jerked under my feet and spun beneath me. I was falling right off the face of the earth. Nothing was holding me down. *I will fall right off the earth and into the sky and out into space,* I thought. *I will be gone forever and ever.* I gasped.

With a rush, I remembered. This was not the first time that I had felt this way. The pink cardigan, the lipstick, the police car, the family portrait with Maggie and her triangle ears. It all came rushing back. My first day of kindergarten came roaring through my senses, and I remembered being four years old and walking stiffly and alone, afraid to turn my head, and determined to look like I knew where I was going.

I could still see the policeman, his face stern and his eyes hidden behind his reflective sunglasses. I could hear the chatter of the police radio and the terror of the ride home in a squad car when Mom never showed up at the end of that very first kindergarten day. I could feel the blows landing, *bam bam bam bam,* after I said, "I was scared. I cried."

Standing on that deserted road, I was six years old, and I

knew that I was lost on purpose. I also knew that if I never came home, my mother would revel in the attention that situation would bring. The fake crying, the pretend sobs; I had seen it all before. I heard her voice: "Once is an accident. Twice is on purpose."

I splintered into fury. All my instinctive cautious silence was consumed in the fireball of terror and agonizing hurt. I drew a huge breath and I shrieked into the empty fields.

"Mommy!" The sound ripped through my throat and hurt my ears. I screamed louder. "Mommy!"

I wanted her and I hated her at the exact same moment.

"Where are you? Mommy!" I screamed with fury and terror, standing motionless.

"Mommy!" I turned then, screaming in all directions. "Mommy! Where are you?" My throat was raw, and I screamed with everything I had into the aloneness. Nobody heard. Nobody saw.

"Mommy! Where are you?" My voice was hoarse and my face was hot and sticky. I was bad. I was lost. I did not come straight home. I didn't know how to get home. Empty fields surrounded me. My hair felt straight up and my throat burned.

There was no one. I was no one. I couldn't feel the ground through my worn-out shoes. I was flying away into far, far away now. No one would find me. No one would help me. Nobody loved me. Nobody cared.

I took a deep breath through my raw and burning throat and balled my fists, ready to shriek down the empty mountainside again.

Someone took my right hand. I felt the lightest possible breath of sensation whispering on my palm and wrapping my fingers. I felt the gentle arm as it touched my sleeve on the inside of my wrist. Out of the farthest corner of my right eye I could see colorless motion, indistinct, a vibration maybe, or a blur impossible to see if I turned my head, but clearly standing beside me in the very furthest edges of my vision. I could feel the presence more than I could see it. They were tall and very thin;

a grown-up.

"Steady."

It was not a sound. It was not a word. It was not a touch.

I froze, silent.

My feet were on the ground again in my tight patent-leather shoes, dull gray and worn so thin I could feel the gravel right through the soles.

Years later my therapist would tell me I conjured an older version of myself to keep me company. I smiled and nodded, but I didn't tell her that my slender visitor was distinctly and clearly male.

I stood there, suddenly calmer, and then I heard a car coming from behind. A shiny white sedan pulled up beside me. It looked fancy and expensive. The passenger window rolled down and a man with white hair and rosy cheeks smiled at me.

"Hey there! Are you lost?" He was nicely dressed in a white dress shirt and a blue-and-red-striped tie.

The hand on mine pulled slightly.

"No," I lied, adjusting my lunch box. "I'm just mad." I quickly wiped my tears with the other hand. The man smiled again. His face was red and shiny against the silvery white hair, the white shirt, and the white car.

"Okay. But you look like you are lost. I can give you a ride if you want."

I felt the hand tugging me backwards, away from the car. I backed away. "No, thank you. I'm not lost." Briskly I started walking forward.

"Okay. Suit yourself." He rolled up the window and the car pulled smoothly and quietly past me. I turned and watched it disappear over the next hill.

I was not alone. We passed another construction site, more plastic sheets loosely blowing in the breeze. It was also empty. I wondered if I should try to find a hiding place there and wait for a police car to come by. I remembered the other policeman in Darien when I was four.

Morgan Hill was a donkey-stripe road of cow pastures and

unfinished houses. Emily was long gone and so was her house. I turned to look for her, but there was nothing. I thought about going back to her house, but I had to go straight home. That was the rule.

I looked again at the blowing plastic of the house up ahead. I could see right through the walls of the frame of this house, and I decided there was nowhere there to hide. No other cars came. It would be a long time before a police car might come by. I pictured myself alone in the empty skeleton ghost house at night, and I kept walking.

The red-faced man came back again, promising candy and phone calls and dinner and cookies and ice cream and puppies, and again that breath of motion, just out of reach of the corner of my eye, whispered up my right arm and tugged me away further off the shoulder, out of reach.

"No thanks," I called. "I'm fine."

The third time, the red-faced man had the window down in his car as he pulled alongside me. Sweat beaded on his forehead, and a drop slid down the side of his purpling face.

"I know you're lost," he whispered. "Why don't you get in the car and come home with me?"

In the distance, a blue car glided over the hill towards us. It looked far, far away. I saw it turn into the driveway of the house on my left. Every fiber of my body wanted to get to that faraway car.

"You can have some ice cream and we'll call the police. They will help you find your mom."

"No, thanks!" I shouted. "That's my mom's car right there!"

I sprinted down Lakeview Drive, my Scooby-Doo lunch box banging against my leg. I felt my arms pumping and the gravel on the shoulder slippery underfoot. I ran, my feet sore on the soles now from the gravel, sharp under the thin, worn-out soles of my shoes. I could feel my feet slapping the asphalt through the thin soles. My lungs gasped for air. The red-faced man's car was still beside me.

In the distance, I saw a woman get out of her car and walk

around her garage to the right. I ran up the hill and past the mailbox on the left. My lungs burned and I gasped as the gravel shot like marbles beneath my soles. I slid around the mailbox and pounded down the driveway.

Behind me I heard the quiet engine of the white sedan accelerate louder, and then fade away. My side ached as I ran to the concrete steps on the right side of the house. I tripped going up the stairs and scraped my palm on the rough edge. I scrambled up the last steps on all fours, and I clenched my burning palm into a fist. I rang the doorbell, panting and clutching my side, with my fiery fist pressed into the stitch in my side.

The door opened right away.

"Yes?" A skinny lady in a skirt and blouse frowned at me.

"I'm lost." My breath gasped out of me. A bigger cramp pinched my side, and I grabbed my stomach and coughed. "I don't know how to get home."

Something was wrong with my eyes. They were wet. I coughed again. My throat hurt from screaming. The cramp in my side finally started to ease, and I stood up straighter and wiped at my eyes with my scraped-up hand. The tears burned the skin, and I wiped my palm on my jeans in the same place that I'd wiped the spit that morning.

My hair felt like freezing ice water on my head. I wanted to run away from the lady, but behind me was spinning lostness, so I forced myself to stand still, caught in the middle between two unknown terrors. The lady tilted her head and looked at me, frowning.

"I'm lost," I said again. My front half wanted to run to her, my back half wanted to run screaming away. I rocked back and forth on my feet, ready to run for it. She opened the door again another crack wider and looked at me with narrow eyes; at my lunch box and my windbreaker.

"Aren't you a little old to be lost?"

Gravity

I rocked back on my heels, gravity loosening its fragile grip on me. I clenched the handle of my lunch box tight in my injured hand and shouted, "I'm just tall!" Tears fell down the front of my T-shirt, leaving wet tracks. "You're a mean lady!"

Away! Away, away, my body shrieked. I backed away, turning sideways, getting ready to run for it.

"I'm only six! I'm just tall!" I shouted, angry tears falling down.

The wild sensation of falling off the world returned, and my ice water hair ran all over my arms and legs. The mean lady drew back slightly into her house. I inhaled.

"Mommy! I want my mommy!" I screamed as loud as I could, the sound ripping through my hoarse, raw throat. I spun around there on the concrete, shrieking. "Mommy! Where are you!"

"Okay. It's okay." The mean lady opened the door all the way, her eyes wide and concerned now. She waved her arms soothingly. "Don't worry, it's all right. What happened?"

Sobbing, I told her everything. She asked me what my address was, and then my phone number. I didn't know, because no one had taught me. Something about her eyes changed then.

"You don't know where you live or your phone number?" She watched me carefully as she handed me a tissue from the box on the table by the door.

"No. I just know our house is yellow with brown trim."

"What day did you move here?"

"On Saturday."

"Two days ago?" She stood straighter and watched me carefully.

"Uh huh."

We drove around for a long time. In the car I told the nice lady about my first day of kindergarten in Darien, and how my mom hadn't shown up at pickup time that day. I cried as I told the lady how my mom hadn't shown up on my first day of school in San Jose, either. She asked questions and listened. Suddenly I saw the yellow house, hidden in its valley.

The nice lady with straight hair slowed down and turned into the driveway. She carefully drove down the long, steep zigzagging slope of the winding driveway and parked the car on the snake head at the bottom. She got out, walked around the car, and opened the door for me. We walked together to the front door.

My body tilted towards the door to go home, and then away. I wobbled on my worn-out Mary Janes. It was weird to stand outside the front door like company and wait for someone to let me in. I felt the spinning vastness of the universe touch my back and the chattering fear of the monster in the house waiting. I vacillated between the monster I knew and the monsters unknown. The nice lady rang the doorbell.

Mom opened the door and I dodged past her to the right and then ran up the eight stairs to my room. Angry voices chased me to my room, but my ears didn't listen. I shut the door and my ears and my heart and my eyes and my tears and my fists and I hid under my new Marimekko butterfly comforter.

I won't listen to the words, or the loud, angry shouts. I was bad. I didn't go straight home. I deserved what I got. Like my first day of kindergarten, I didn't get dinner. At bedtime she limped into my room.

"Why do you always have to cause so much trouble?" Her face was stern in the dim light. "I told you to come straight home." She emphasized the words dramatically: *Straight. Home.* She tapped my nose on both words. I lay, frozen, not breathing. Her mouth turned down, pouty.

"This is all your fault," she said in her Whiny Little Girl voice. She thrust her lower lip out, large, her eyes sad. She put both hands up over her heart. "That lady hurt my feelings." Baby Talk voice. Then, eyes hard and tight, in her You're in Trouble voice she scolded, "You embarrassed me today."

She glared at me though her clear cat eyeglasses. I didn't dare breathe. She chucked me under the chin and grinned a great big mean grin. I felt my hands shaking under the thick new yellow comforter. I twisted the matching sheet anxiously, pressing the roll of sheet up to my chin.

"I'm sorry, Mommy." I said, my eyes prickling. I tried desperately to stop the tears. "I tried to come straight home. I didn't know how."

"You are so stupid!" She jabbed me hard with her finger in my leg. "A big girl like you should know how to get home." She jabbed me hard twice more on the words "big girl," and then again on "home." I pulled my leg away as far as I was able without moving my torso.

"I'm sorry, Mommy," I pleaded. I couldn't hold back the tears anymore. "Why didn't you come to the bus stop, Mommy?"

Her reaction was immediate. She pulled back away from me, her back straight and her big eyes stretched wide. "I had to make the kids a snack. I couldn't come to the bus stop just for you." She said it *youuuuuuuuwah!*

"I was scared. I wanted you to be there. I wanted you to help me."

"Well, I couldn't. Your sister wanted cheese and crackers."

A few weeks later, the lady from DCFS showed up, which only made it worse.

***

"When do I get to take algebra?" Sebastian cried, his little toddler body flung against my shoulder.

I juggled the bag of Goldfish crackers in one hand and tried to calm my sobbing toddler on my shoulder with the other. I was standing in the parking lot at preschool drop-off, and my three-year-old was wailing on my shoulder like his heart was going to break. I wondered how Sebastian even knew the word algebra. It was probably his teenage babysitter, I realized, but that still didn't explain the heartrending toddler tears every day over math. In high school, I cried for the day I could stop taking math, and I wondered for the millionth time, whose child was this, and where was mine?

I had no idea what to do for Sebastian's preschool algebra obsession. It will be one of my regrets that I didn't just simply teach it to him. At the time, I felt incompetent in that regard. We live in a society where everyone is categorized. I had my niche, my role, my label: Music teacher, mother, wife. Algebra teacher was out of my realm, even for a three-year-old. Now in hindsight, I think how ridiculous that I felt I needed a degree to just do the math.

I truly felt math-incompetent, though, and so I did what any self-respecting music teacher would do. I knew that music and math are related, so perhaps piano would fill some of the longing. We already had Musikgarten classes once a week with Sebastian's beloved Miss Caryn Borgetti, so piano felt like a natural addition. I found a wonderful private teacher who was willing to work with Sebastian the next year at the age of four because he was already reading.

I bought a book about raising a gifted child, which proved to be very affirming. Gifted children often have anxiety, I learned. They are more aware of danger and death at a very young age. According to the book, gifted children often find moving stressful. Sebastian's "I'm Nervous Game" and the algebra crying started shortly after we bought the new house. Everything clicked.

Life went on happily. Sebastian loved preschool, his teacher, and his best friend there, even without the desired algebra, but he still cried at drop-off. The moms of the confident toddlers consoled each other because their children ran into the classroom without a backwards glance. Those moms felt the sweet success of social confidence with the sting of no longer being needed quite so much. We moms of criers gave them envious glances and consoled each other that our children would eventually grow out of it. Sebastian and I made friends with another drop-off crier, Jason, and his lovely mom, Lily.

Jason and Sebastian both had a lot of imagination and got on well together. We were at Jason's house the day the two four-year-olds decided to take the training wheels off their bikes.

Jason got the balance first, and Sebastian was almost there when it was time to go home for lunch. Sebastian couldn't wait for lunch to be over before trying again. When we finished, I walked it for him down the driveway to the quiet cul-de-sac and steadied the bike for him as he climbed on.

Almost immediately, he had it. I jogged behind him for just a few steps, and then his back straightened. I could see the subtle wobble as his body found its center of gravity. He leaned slightly, and he and his bike followed the curve of the black asphalt in a large ring.

"Don't stop pedaling!" I called, paralyzed between chasing after him and just letting him go. He picked up speed and I stopped, clutching my hands anxiously and waiting for the inevitable spill. It didn't happen.

Sebastian tilted his body to the left, and the bike wobbled again. I flinched and suddenly his center of balance restored. He pedaled around and around the cul-de-sac. I stood in the center, my breath blown out of me. And then he sang, the only song he has ever sung to me. I hear it always in the background when I remember this shining moment, his triumph and his joy ringing through the clear day.

"I took off my training wheels, so appa dacka shpayniels!"

His voice was a true and clear soprano, joyous and proud. He sang the words in that typical sol-mi-la pattern so common in young singers. Mi sol sol sol la sol sol, sol mi sol sol sol la sol sol.

In my mind's eye I still see him, the king of the universe. He is laughing. He is capable. The breeze lifts his blond hair and he tests the strength of his legs as he pedals. He sings his joy as he loops around the black universe of asphalt. My heart flies with him as the gravity that binds us together weakens. He expands his orbit, his small sneakered feet whirring in their own double planetary system.

Sebastian's hands hold tightly to the handlebars. The front wheel shakes tentatively and then straightens as he finds the obliquity of his balance. He leans around the curve of his circumgyration, singing and pedaling, his feet turning sidereal beats to the music. His elbows are rings and he is flying free.

Kindergarten

"Hey! Look at me! I'm on the monkey bars!"

Sebastian was flying one-armed from the first bar on the jungle gym. We had just finished kindergarten orientation, and now all the kids were running around the playground. His kindergarten teacher had looked a little harried and frazzled, but her smile was genuine and warm during her presentation. As she went on about phonics, I had written the expected love note and drawn a heart.

"Dear Sebastian, Happy first day of kindergarten! I love you so much! Love, Mom."

I drew a big, lopsided heart around the words and put XXXXs and OOOOs for hugs and kisses underneath where I signed "Mom." The teacher collected the letters from each parent to surprise the children with the next day. They would each receive a note from home to remind them they were loved. Mrs. Buckles had been doing this for a while and had it down.

Now all the kids were running madly around the playground. Sebastian made a grab for the next bar after the closest one and caught it. He swung his legs, trying to get the momentum to skip another bar. He didn't quite have the swing in his pelvis just right to make the grab for the bar, so he missed. Swinging one-armed, he flailed for a moment and then dropped to the ground. He landed lightly, first feet then hands, in the thick wood chips. He brushed his hands off as he turned to me, face alight.

"Watch me! I'm going to do it again!" He ran around to the ladder and waited his turn.

At home Sebastian asked for a bedtime snack. Over homemade chocolate chip cookies, Sebastian asked what algebra was.

I looked at him.

"Algebra is where you substitute a letter N for the value of a number, like this." I wrote 3 + N = 5 on his napkin with a red marker.

"That's easy. N is two," he said matter-of-factly, then took another bite of his cookie.

Eric and I exchanged an amused glance.

"Try this one," I suggested, and wrote 8 + N = 3.

Sebastian laughed. "That's easy! N is minus-5."

Eric and I looked at each other again and laughed.

"How does he know negatives?" Eric asked.

"I don't know." I thought a moment, and then remembered. "But he was asking to buy a toy the other day and I told him that he had spent all of his allowance." To Sebastian, I said, "And I already lent you extra to buy the last toy." We grinned silly grins at each other and touched noses. "I told him that he had negative allowance."

Sebastian and I exchanged a look. He smirked. I smirked back with a silly face. "When he asked what negative allowance means, I told him that it means he owes me money," I growled, mock threatening. Sebastian leaned away, laughing.

"Mom!"

"When he asked how much, I drew him a number line."

Eric nodded at Sebastian with pride. "Pretty clever!" They high-fived.

"I owe three dollars!" Sebastian announced happily to Eric. "I have minus-three dollars. Can I have another cookie?" I passed him the small one on my plate.

"Thank you!" He cheered and dunked it in his milk.

***

I dipped my strawberry in my champagne and took a bite at the Cheers or Tears party the next morning. The ripe berry was floral and sweet against the dry champagne as I put the green top down on my plate and reached for another one. My hand was jittery as I pulled a small red berry from the lovely platter.

"Your husband has a really big deck," a familiar, sly voice whispered in my ear.

I snorted as I turned, champagne stinging my sinus cavities

and bringing tears to my eyes. My girlfriend stood, one hand on hip, her eyes flashing wickedly. She was a natural mimic.

"Stop," I whispered, my eyes stinging. "Unless you want this on you." I waved my champagne glass in her direction.

She grinned at me, her thick, pale hair neatly bumped into an elegant ponytail. We were both dressed nicely for my first and her fourth back-to-school Tears or Cheers party, but her hourglass figure looked especially elegant in her dark jeans and nice top.

"Are you cheering or tearing?" she asked.

"Some of both," I shrugged, hoping that I was hiding my tears successfully. "You?"

"The same," she said, with a sympathetic smile.

I felt a surge of gratitude for this nonjudgmental friend. We smiled and chatted.

On the walk home from the Cheers or Tears party, I thought about the events of the morning. I made Sebastian's first day of kindergarten completely unlike my own, in every single way that I could make it. First thing, before Sebastian was even up, I set my oven timer for twenty minutes before pickup time.

Sebastian got to pick out his favorite outfit and we laughed together as I did his hair special in the morning with a touch of gel. I gave him a Mohawk, and he giggled at himself in the mirror, then smashed it down.

"That's silly, Mom!"

I made him his favorite pancakes and bacon for breakfast. Then we gathered up his brand-new backpack and took pictures at the door, and again with his friend down the street. Together we walked cheerfully the couple of blocks to the school. I snapped a great picture of the two of them standing outside the school doors. In the photo, Sebastian smiled with so much mischief beside his friend.

"I love you, Mama," he said.

"I love you, too. Have a great day today, and I'll see you at lunchtime." I hugged him and kissed his cheek. I smoothed his hair and caught another mom's eyes over his head. Her son was clinging, but not crying. A surge of empathy welled up inside me for her.

"Have a great day, honey. I love you. I'll see you very soon!" I gave Sebastian a gentle push.

"Bye, Mom."

The friendly assistant swept him in, kindly but no-nonsense.

After the Cheers or Tears party I went home and did my chores. Folding laundry, my anxiety rose. I tried feeling my feelings, but that only made it worse. I tried distraction. The sense of danger rose as I went about my day mopping and cleaning. *Be kind to yourself*, I reminded myself for the hundredth time. Anyone who survived your childhood would feel anxious today.

Mentally, I reviewed the list of friends in the neighborhood that I could call if I had some unplanned emergency and I couldn't get back to school to pick up Sebastian. First, there was Eric. Then I had three friends close by whom I trusted completely; four more in a pinch. If all else failed I could call the school if something happened.

I looked around my tidy house. I had vacuumed, dusted, and mopped. I felt silly. I'd been picking Sebastian up on time for two years at preschool, without a hitch. What could possibly happen?

***

My herbal tea smelled refreshingly citrusy as I sat down to take a short break. The house was tidy and the laundry was folded. I sipped my tea and read the newspaper, glad for a few minutes to myself. The kitchen timer went off, bringing me back to the present with a jolt.

Sebastian. I had to go and pick him up from kindergarten. I freshened my makeup and checked my hair before putting on my sneakers and walking the few blocks to the school. I was the first one there, at least ten minutes early.

The dismissal process at Sebastian's school was an exercise in military precision. Orange cones and signs on the lawn waited for the outgoing crowd. The school bell blasted, and the shouts of imaginary children cascaded around me as the real children filed out in quiet, orderly lines. I couldn't help comparing it to the chaos of my own first day of kindergarten. I remembered the shouting and shoving, feral frenzy of school dismissal in the early 1970s.

Mobs of screaming children, unchecked by any adults, cascaded through my mind's eye. In my remembered crowd, my four-year-old self is lost. Standing there waiting for Sebastian's class to come out, I remembered the woman with the blonde French twist and the black cat eyeglasses who had looked so much like my own mother that I ran towards her, wondering where she had gotten the new clothes.

I remembered the shock I felt after the lady bent down to hug another little girl; only then did I realize she wasn't my own mother. I remembered the hurt and anger I felt when I saw that my mother was the only mother who hadn't come. I understood the wrongness at age four.

I remember turning to look for my teacher, and seeing she was gone. I can still see the angle of the light as the hours went by while I waited outside the school, alone. I remember dropping my crumpled family portrait on the sidewalk when I finally went looking for my mother, thinking she was lying on the sidewalk somewhere, hurt and needing my help.

I remember the stiffness in my spine and neck as I walked, afraid to turn my head. I could still picture the police officer's unsmiling face, his eyes hidden behind the aviator-style sunglasses, and the sound of the radio in the squad car. I could hear my mother's voice as I slipped between her and the doorway and ran past her to hide in the family room.

"Are you calling me a bad mother?" She whipped her most patrician tones out at the policeman. "How dare you."

These memories coursed through me as I stood in front of Sebastian's school with the other parents. I watched as the teachers escorted their charges out in perfect, silent single-file lines. They arranged themselves in predetermined columns in the grass with little signs announcing the teachers' names and grade levels at the front.

I watched the procession of students eagerly with the other parents, searching for Sebastian's face and feeling the same overwhelming love for him and simultaneous incredulity at the enormity of my mother's illness. Sebastian's teacher led her little soldiers to their places and checked off each parent by name on her class list before handing each child over.

Sebastian was laughing with the boy beside him. The two swatted at each other playfully. I greeted Mrs. Buckles and then waved, calling, "Sebastian!" The motion of my hand and the sound of my voice in the crowd drew his attention. He smiled and ran to me.

"Mama!"

I knelt down and caught him.

***

"Hey, kiddo! How was your first day?"

He leaned into my hug, his fine hair brushing my chin. I squeezed him lightly and kissed the back of his head, his short, dark blond hair silky against my lips.

"Fine." He pulled away from the hug and smiled brilliantly in the afternoon sun.

"What did you do?" He wiggled out of my grasp and I slid him down to the grass.

"Phonics." He shrugged. "What are we having for lunch?"

"Mac and cheese or leftover pot roast. You pick."

"Mac and cheese!" His eyes glowed as brilliantly as his smile. "Can we play badminton first?"

"For a few minutes, sure."

We walked home companionably, and I quickly strung the badminton net up across the driveway.

I passed him the blue racquet and ducked under the net to the other side. "Better watch out! Here comes the first shot." I whacked a high shot over the net, and it sailed into the center of the court.

"I got it!" Sebastian slapped the birdie back over to me.

"What was the best thing that happened to you today?" I missed an easy return, ran and picked up the birdie, and served it again, this time crookedly. Sebastian ran into the grass to return it and missed.

"Badminton!" He shouted and served the birdie back to me and hit the net. He ran and untangled it, and served another one, an easy shot.

"I meant at kindergarten, silly." I managed to return the birdie, and we volleyed back and forth.

"Recess. I dunno." Sebastian slapped the birdie hard with his racquet. "Look, Mom! That one went right through the basketball hoop!"

The days and weeks turned into months and every day it was the same. Sebastian would not talk about school. He was such a happy kid at home. Every trip to Walmart or Meijer he danced down the aisle, both arms out. He twirled and leaped in exuberance and played hours of pretend battles against dragons, Snape and Voldemort. He made lots and lots of art. I couldn't keep up with all the art. He talked non stop about everything he saw and did at home or with friends, but I never heard a peep about his life at school.

I felt like a trial lawyer who had a serious crush on a hostile witness.

"What was the best thing that happened today?" Or "What made you sad today at school?"

"Nothing," he said. Then he looked at me with annoyance and sighed. "Can I read now?" Or "Can I draw now?"

My mother passed away in February, and over the next eighteen months I lost more than one hundred pounds. The weight melted away easily, along with the fear and anger, after her passing. I kept my promise to Sebastian, and I never let her see or touch him. Restricting carbs and working out six days a week had worked. I lost a person, in weight and life, both life-threateningly unhealthy. I met my ideal weight on October 27,

2009, and I kept those pounds off easily for eight years, three months, and eleven days.

Astrology and Astronomy

I sang a song about sex at my mother's funeral. Actually, it was at her internment in Canada, about four months after she passed away from lung cancer. After years of smoking, the cancer had colonized her lungs aggressively, and then, perhaps inspired by the wanderlust of their generous hostess, decided to migrate to bonier homes, where it multiplied rapidly. It was an honest mistake; the song, not the cancer.

The cancer was the result of years of cultivation of poison, both inhaled and expulsed phonetically, with many long-aspirated vowels. My mother had swum for years through poisoned vapors of her own exhalations, and I think the cancer knew it had found a commodious and accommodating host that brewed murderous and terrifying statements. It is always the words that kill or save you.

I wonder now... if I had known just how much words would save Sebastian, what could I have done differently? There are a few things, like the algebra; that's a fact. Overall, I think I did well, accidentally; like I did for my mom at her internment, but for entirely different reasons. I calculate that my mom would have been secretly thrilled about her inappropriate but gorgeous musical sendoff; a love song for a woman who couldn't love me. She was an atheist who loved bombastic music, and she would have reveled in the soaring Gwyneth Walker melody with its explosive vocal climax.

Now that I know Scorpio is the sign of passion, the fact that I didn't get the references in the song to oars and rowing boats, or to the earth and deep roots, is pretty funny. I do love a good metaphor. I interpreted the poet May Swenson's line "*Burn radiant love, born scorpion need*" to mean a burning sting of Cupid's arrow. I didn't know my own astrological characteristics. I could not do the math, so to speak.

Calculating how many words saved Sebastian is a different math, like counting the stars. It's a form of visual-spatial intelligence, if you will pardon the pun. We stand, rods and cones, under the star-soaked parasol of infinity, photons dripping liquid spark-rain through our corneal atmosphere until we are too electrically dazzled to do the algebra. What does N equal in infinity? A single letter, floating in chaos, perhaps; nothing more.

***

Sebastian flew through kindergarten and first grade with perfect marks and nice friends, but he never grew more talkative about it. He did meet his best friend at the neighborhood block party the summer before second grade. Sebastian had spent the past two hours painting his face with one design after another. I could smell the tang of the face paint when he popped up from under the folding table he'd been hiding under.

"Roaaahhhr!" he growled. "I'm a tiger!" He looked more like a zombie with the layers of paint all blurred together, but whatever. I cringed back in mock fear and shrieked obligingly, and then with my cat's paws I reached out to swipe back at him.

A new family had just arrived, with a little girl Sebastian's age. A nice family with two working parents, we chatted. They had just moved back to the neighborhood after living out of state for several years. Their daughter was beautifully dressed in a perfectly pressed sundress, her short brown bob framing her heart-shaped face.

This new little girl was so polite and had such beautiful manners. Somehow these two opposites hit it off. They didn't see each other again until the first day of second grade. The way April tells it, she recognized Sebastian first.

"Wait," April said. "Weren't you at the block party?"

And that was it. They were best friends, inseparable.

April's friendship was pure joy for Sebastian. What April lacked in height she made up for in determination and spirit. The two friends rode bikes together all around the neighborhood and to the park. They planned multi day sleepovers and camping trips. We took April camping at Kankakee State Park, and we all brought our bikes.

The bike trails ran for miles along the Kankakee River. Neat green grass lined the path and old tall trees sheltered us with their shade in cool puddles of deeper green. The river loped over boulders and stones, making a bubbling counterpoint to the trees' chordal harmonies. The whir of our tires on the asphalt path made a three-part motet of peace.

Sebastian had just graduated to his first geared bike. It was a ten-speed and it was almost too big for his tall frame and long legs. I wanted it to last a while. April had brought her Disney princess bike, the one she had quite grown out of. April had to pedal like mad to keep up with us. Side by side, these two kids looked miles apart, but they were twins inside.

At playdates, every single toy Sebastian owned was strewn across the basement floor in elaborate make-believe scenarios. They played *Robinson Crusoe* and *Island of the Blue Dolphins* and spent many hours hiding out in the play forts they build in the backyard with ropes and blankets. April practically lived at our home, and the two kids entertained each other for days at a time, without fighting. I never once had to settle a dispute. April became part of our family.

One weekend we packed the tent and we went, just the three of us, to Rock Cut State Park in Rockford. After sunset we walked across the dim parking lot to a large field. Lightning bugs signaled. The clear purple sky deepened to indigo blue as we walked through the gloaming gray grasses. Night drew its curtains across the stage of sky, and the invisible spotlight of the sun flamed across Venus, low on the horizon.

The old rhyme "Star light, star bright, the first star I see tonight; I wish I may, I wish I might, have the wish I wish tonight" teased my memory. I looked at my two shadowed wishes, standing hand in hand beside me, and I reached for Eric's other hand. We waited.

A telescope was mounted on a concrete platform, and a local astronomer wearing chinos and a polo shirt chatted softly with the assembled campers. The sky darkened to soft blue-black and the hush of wind in the grass was the breath of an expectant audience. The gathered families whispered and were silent, watching.

A star appeared in the dark sky, and as always, I heard Richard Hundley at his superlunary piano play a pianissimo C#. And then, one by one cantabile, the other stars appeared, as though each was individually spotlit; each star was a note. A liquid scrim fell across the star-sound sky as the notes became a pageant of whirling dancers caught in a resplendent slow motion pavane.

Almost invisible in the dark, Eric turned towards me and kissed me softly. The astronomer gestured at the brilliant peerage in the clear and still deepening night and asked if anyone knew how to find a constellation.

"I do!" Sebastian raised his hand, almost invisibly in the starlight dim.

The volunteer astronomer replied cheerfully, "Which one?"

"There's Gemini!" Sebastian pointed to the argent sky, wheeling with brilliant pinpoint suns; my seven-year-old astronomer. I have only ever been able to find Orion with any reliability, and my eyebrows shot up in the dark.

"How does he know where Gemini is?" I whispered to Eric.

"I showed him a couple years ago."

The astronomer laughed and handed Sebastian his laser pointer. "Show everyone where it is."

"Well," Sebastian said, aiming his laser into the ceaseless deep, "it's right there, by those two stars. That star is Castor and this other one is Pollux. Gemini means twins."

***

Sebastian and April formed an extraordinary friendship. The complex universe they invented manifested as a galaxy of toys pinwheeled across the basement floor. Because their games had complex storylines that grew over time, and my out-of-sight, out-of-mind hierarchy of cleaning priorities, I left them there.

Sebastian auditioned for the school talent show in third grade and made it. The old school piano could not be moved onto the stage for his performance, and so it was arranged on the gym floor at the front and to the left side of the stage, out of range of any stage lights. At the performance, there was a glitch with the spotlight, so he played his Kuhlau sonatina completely in the dark, from memory.

Sebastian rocked his entrance, walked out like he owned the place, gave everyone a big smile, and then settled himself at the piano. The gym lights went out, the spot failed to come on, then off he went, without a hitch. He played beautifully, with lovely technique and expression. He played the scales running up and down, each note ringing clearly on the old school piano.

There was one minor bobble when he got off track with his right hand. He didn't play a wrong note, but just forgot what notes came next. He vamped the Alberti bass for a measure and then came right back in, both hands spotlessly. The one measure addition was imperceptible to anyone who didn't know the piece.

Afterwards, I congratulated Sebastian on a fine performance and asked him how he felt about playing in the dark. He shrugged and smiled. "It's no big deal."

"You played beautifully. I'm so proud of you. Did it bother you when the spotlight didn't come on?"

"No, not really. I didn't need it anyway."

April ran up beaming, hugged him, and congratulated him. "Great job, Sebastian!"

And they were off and running all around the gym with all the other kids.

***

On a bitter cold day in December, Karla Cossa, Sebastian's third-grade gifted teacher, came running out the door of the school without a coat on, calling my name and flagging me down, quickly telling me her news. I stared at her in shock, feeling the icy wind pushing the hood of my parka back, and gasped.

"What? Are you kidding me? When did he do this?"

"Yeah. He didn't tell you?" Karla's lovely eyes searched mine, concerned. She shivered in the winter wind.

"Karla, you know he doesn't tell me anything." I sighed. "He talks all day long about everything else, but he never says a word about what goes on at school. I have to eavesdrop on his friends and stalk their moms to find out anything about what goes on during the day."

Karla frowned, and then smiled at me. "Well, he finished the fourth-grade math book first quarter. We can't meet his needs at this level. He needs to move up."

Sebastian was in third grade, and he had never been coached or tutored in math. I stood there in the freezing wind, acutely aware of how many families would be thrilled to get this news. Everything is so competitive in our society, and I knew parents who pushed for grade promotion, often for kids who would be terribly served by it. I was devastated, and Karla looked at me kindly. She had been designing special pull-out programs specifically for Sebastian's academic needs since he was in kindergarten. She was very dedicated, and I knew she had Sebastian's best interests at heart.

My mother had tried to effectively double promote me when I was seven. She enrolled me in a special gifted class called Kleinschule in Morgan Hill. The class was designed for gifted fourth-through-sixth graders. She convinced the teacher to take me as a third grader, when I was already the youngest one in my class with my November birthday. I remember just wanting to play with kids my own age on the playground, and so I refused to do the work and got sent back to my beloved third grade teacher about a month later. At least one of us made good decisions.

While Sebastian had several good friends in third grade, he didn't have any friends in the grade above. Although our school was only a few blocks away, the vast majority of the children who attended the school were bused in from a neighboring town. The children from our small neighborhood made only a tiny percentage of the student body. I didn't want to separate him from his friends, especially April.

I had built an iron wall of protection around Sebastian because I had no other choice. I was proud of it. Only safe people crossed my protective gate and I was unapologetic about it. If I didn't like children or their parents, they weren't welcomed in. My creep detector was highly refined. I didn't want to start the friends process over.

At the school meeting I voiced all those concerns and then we talked about Sebastian's educational level and needs. The gifted math instructor was curious.

"I gave him the fifth-grade math assessment. What I can't figure out is how he knew how to multiply and divide fractions."

I was speechless. I cleared my throat and shook my head. "I have no idea."

I looked at Eric, who was sitting quietly, looking thoughtful. His eyes brightened, and he laughed. "Oh, he asked about it once last year, so I showed him."

We explained our concerns about the grade promotion, and Eric and I asked for alternatives. We were given three choices, all with serious drawbacks. We could bus Sebastian to the middle school for math, but he would be the only one going, and he would miss forty minutes of instruction every day due to travel time. Sebastian was adamant about not wanting to be the only kid riding a bus to the middle school for math, and none of us wanted him to miss art and music and who knew what else every day. We rejected that proposal.

The school counselor then told us that the only other option was "Independent Study" for math. Sebastian would go to the library by himself every day for math time, they told us, faces mask-like. When I asked who would be overseeing this "independent study," they couldn't tell me who, or if anyone would be assigned. I thought about my own experience with independent study for AP French 4 my senior year of high school. The only section of that class conflicted with madrigal choir, so I and one of the altos took regular French and got AP credit doing extra assignments.

Madame sent the two of us to the library everyday to keep our bored hijinks from interfering with her Je vais à la plage-ing. I mentally pictured Sebastian, age eight, sneaking onto the Metra and escaping to Sportsman's Park. We rejected independent study for Sebastian, as there were also no accommodations for his verbal giftedness.

It was apparent that grade promotion was the least bad of the three choices for Sebastian, despite our concerns about his friendships. The next step in the process was IQ testing. At the office before the IQ testing, the psychologist asked the purpose for the test. I explained about Sebastian finishing the fourth-grade math book without help, the choices we'd been offered by the school, and our reasons for acquiescing to the grade promotion, imperfect as it was.

After the testing was completed, Sebastian and I sat down with the psychologist. Sebastian had scored in the ninety-ninth percentile in verbal ability but was only upper average in the visual-spatial.

Surprised, I asked, "What does that mean?" I gestured at the comparatively low visual-spatial scores. "Sebastian is excellent at math. I thought that visual-spatial abilities are associated with math ability."

"They are," the psychologist agreed. "It means he's slower at processing math."

"But he's not slower at processing math. He finished the fourth-grade math book first quarter, and no one coached him."

"Ummhmm." She made a note in her file.

"Sebastian learned to multiply and divide fractions from being shown one time, a year ago. He's never had any practice since."

"I see." She glanced at Sebastian and looked down at her papers again.

"I don't understand why there is such a big gap in his scores."

She looked up. "It means he's slower at processing math."

"But he's not slower at math, he's faster," I said, feeling

annoyance rise. “That makes no sense.”

The psychologist looked me in the eyes, her face a mask. “It means he’s not as smart as you think he is.”

Potted Plant

The school administration pushed us to promote Sebastian into fourth grade after winter break. Eric and I refused. We insisted that Sebastian remain in third grade with his friends during the mornings for the remainder of the year. That way he could eat lunch and go to recess with his friends in the morning and also get to know the older fourth graders in the afternoon in the gifted fifth-grade math class. We talked about the choices with Sebastian many times and told him he could choose to stay in his grade with April.

"There's more to life than work," I said, and meant it. "Friendships are important."

Sebastian was eager to move ahead. Together, as a family, we cautiously embarked on the new plan. On the first day back after winter break, Sebastian came home with a brand-new fourth-grade friend we approved of, and then several others. He was still best friends with April, and everything was going great.

In the fall, Sebastian started fifth grade. April's fourth-grade classroom was close by, and all I heard from April was how often she was in Sebastian's classroom. Before school, after school, she was always present, she told me happily. I thought the two friends were together more now than at any other time. I had no idea how the teachers felt about April's invasion of the fifth grade, but as far as I could tell, no one stopped her.

About a week into fifth grade I asked Sebastian, "How was your day?"

Sebastian's blue eyes glowed with excitement. "It was awesome! We are doing the digestive system and reading fractured fairy tales. We are going to get to write our own stories and publish them."

He chattered on and on while I stared at him in shock. Then my tears came pouring down. Sebastian fell silent and his eyes filled with concern. "Why are you crying, Mom?"

"I'm crying because I'm so happy."

He leaned back and crossed his arms, then looked at me like

I was about to put a lampshade on my head and dance the conga. "Why?"

"Today is the first time you have come home from school excited." I brushed the tears from my cheeks. "It's the first time I've seen you come home happy."

Sebastian's eyes were riveted on mine, concerned.

"No matter what I asked you, you wouldn't talk to me about your day. It's the first time you shared with me what happened at school," I explained.

"Well, Mom," he explained slowly and patiently, "that's because a lot of things happened, but none of it was interesting."

I stared at him silently for a long moment. Then the laughter came boiling up. Me first, then Sebastian. We threw back our heads and howled. I slid off the sofa to the beige carpet and Sebastian rolled onto the floor next to me, his soprano peals of laughter mixing with mine. I felt the rough carpet underneath my hands as years of anxious worry lifted off me, evaporating. Gasping for breath, tears and laughter mixed together, I imitated his forceful inflection.

"Well, Mom," I mimicked his professorial tones. "That's because a lot of things happened, but none of it was interesting."

Sebastian was silent for a moment, then he hooted with laughter, rolling on the floor next to me, knees drawn up as he rocked from side to side. Laughter exploded out of me as I lay next to him, watching his joy, seeing his face lit up with hilarity and relief.

Sebastian froze suddenly and then sat up; eyes fierce. I sat up and faced him. He looked me straight in the eyes and spoke from his heart.

"Well... It's true."

His perfect Duesing blue eyes were so serious and wise beyond his years, I was sad and grateful at the same time; sad it took so long for him to get the academic challenge he needed, and grateful we finally had made the right move.

"I am sorry it took so long. I didn't understand how bored you were."

He dove into my arms. He landed hard into my chest, pushing me back against the sofa; his face pressed into the crook of my neck. I was sticky with tears where his face touched my skin.

"I love you, too, Mama. You're the best mom in the world."

***

"All A's and a B in Lit! Congratulations!" I said, feeling sad as I saw his cautious eyes.

Sebastian's newfound joy at school had lasted less than one year. In the spring of fifth grade, Sebastian realized that when he went to middle school, April would not come with him. He grieved as though she were dying. I was devastated for him, and the more we talked about his very real grief, the worse his anxiety and depression became. Always a perfectionist, Sebastian became obsessed with his grades.

Sebastian began to say things like "the world would explode" if he got a B on his report card, and he worried constantly about getting lost at the new school. I was stunned by the sudden change, and quite concerned for my previously very confident son. He had worked himself up into such a state, he seemed terrified of going to middle school. I immediately sought the help of a therapist for him.

The therapist diagnosed Sebastian with anticipational anxiety, and we worked hard to make sure Sebastian knew he was loved and appreciated for the kind, thoughtful, funny person he was. Nothing helped. He seemed to have turned the whole middle school into some kind of terrifying monster.

"You should have seen him," I said to the therapist. "I took him by the middle school to see if we could just do a walk-through before school started, and he was so scared he was sweating. Why would he do that if there wasn't a real fear?"

The therapist explained that with anticipational anxiety, people get better after the event that upsets them occurs.

"Once school starts, he will be fine," she said.

I was concerned and frustrated watching my son's very real distress about a normal life passage, and I didn't know what else to do to help him except to reassure him constantly that everything would be okay. Finally, it was the middle school locker day. Sebastian and I bought all the decorations to make his locker fun and did our back-to-school shopping. We waited in line and picked up his schedule and then went to find his locker. Then we walked his schedule. The school was just a big rectangle and every wing was clearly labeled. We found the library and the art wing right away. We walked his schedule once, then once again.

Just like that, in one day, the anxiety was over. The school year began and Sebastian quickly found his friend group. It was a mixed group of chorus, orchestra, and band kids. They were bright and kind. They adopted April in when she came into the middle school the next year, and the band stayed together all through high school. Best of all, Sebastian got some B's on his report card for the first time ever.

Although the school put everything online so parents could supervise every missing worksheet, Eric and I didn't check on Sebastian ever. He policed himself mercilessly and didn't need any help from me. He watched our reactions carefully with each report card. Sebastian's self-esteem was so wrapped up in this artificial measure of his worth.

One evening Sebastian worried over a math quiz. I offered him help, which he rejected. He said he felt he wasn't prepared enough to get an A and might not get into college because of it. He had always scored in the ninety-ninth percentile on all standardized tests in math and English, without preparation, so I was mystified and sad that he thought a middle school math quiz mattered so much.

I reminded him, for what felt like the thousandth time, that no one ever got rejected from college for not getting an A on a middle school math test. I told him to get as many B's as he wanted. Sebastian was horrified at the idea, but also curious.

We had had this conversation so many times, but it was like this was the first time he had ever heard me. I decided honesty was best. I told him about my high school math triumph my freshman year, savoring the congratulations from that wonderful teacher long ago. I grinned at Sebastian.

"For some reason, I was the only person in the honors algebra group who passed the matrices test on the first try," I bragged. Sebastian nodded at me expectantly. "But the next year I had a terrible teacher for geometry. Every day, he came in and wrote the assignment for the day on the board, and then sat down and read his magazines."

Sebastian nodded again. He knew the type.

"There was no instruction. I mean absolutely none." I leaned forward and put my elbows on my knees. "After every test, he would post the grades on the bulletin board, coded by our ID numbers."

Sebastian listened attentively, not sure where this was going. "What happened?"

"I thought I had done okay on that particular test," I said, humble-bragging about my great achievement in sophomore geometry, "but when I checked my score, I couldn't find it. I kept looking at the list, further and further, and there it was. Finally, I saw it."

Sebastian's eyes were huge. "What did you get, Mom?"

I hesitated, lips pressed together to keep myself from laughing. Sebastian's eyes were so intent, and his forehead wrinkled a little as he watched me. I stilled my face to deliver the news without laughing.

"A four."

Sebastian's forehead knit in confusion. "Out of...?" He tilted his head slightly, questioning.

"A hundred!"

He was slack-jawed with shock. I mashed my lips together to keep myself from laughing and then gave up and laughed anyway.

"And next to my score, in big red letters, do you know what he wrote?" I said, between gasping laughs.

"What?" The horror on his face was awesome.

"Potted Plant.'"

If he had any cavities, I could have counted them. Silence.

He breathed, and then he burst out laughing and I joined him. I straightened up, put my hands on my knees, and I threw down the gauntlet. "Sebastian, I dare you to get a four on tomorrow's math quiz! I dare you."

Sebastian clutched his stomach and rolled from side to side in his chair with his head back. "Oh, my God! Oh, my God!"

"You couldn't do it if you tried," I teased. "Come on. Be a potted plant like your mother."

"Oh my God, Mom!" He howled at the ceiling. He swung both hands up and ruffled his hair, then put his arms down on his legs and laughed at the floor. "The best part is that you thought you did okay."

He was so beautiful, and it made my heart sing to see the anxiety melting away. He was relaxing and having fun. I thought we had this anxiety thing down. Sebastian chose wisely what he wanted to do at school and where he wanted to spend his time. I encouraged him to choose his least interesting classes to slack off in, and he did. His middle school grade reports were sprinkled with a B here and there. Eric and I didn't comment on it, except to say, "Congratulations! Beautiful report card. Where are we going out for dinner?"

***

"I like to do a short ten-minute check-in with my high school patients before bringing the parents back." Dr. Liu's soft red-lipsticked smile was welcoming and friendly. "Is that okay?"

High school was a very welcome change for Sebastian, who appreciated that he had significantly less homework with his all honors and AP class schedule than he had had in middle school. He took as many art classes as he could, where he excelled. He joined the dive and water polo teams, and he chose to get all A's again because he wanted to, not out of fear, and then had gotten a bad concussion in September of his sophomore year in PE.

Sebastian smiled at Dr. Liu, who was dressed in a red-patterned blouse and crisply pressed slacks. "Sure. Thanks."

"I'll be back for you in ten," Dr. Liu said, smiling kindly at me. "This office is a maze."

I used the ten minutes to finish filling out the last two pages of the enormous neuro psych evaluation packet, and I wondered when Sebastian would recover from his concussion. The concussion had set him back for months. It was December now, and Sebastian wasn't improving. He had such severe headaches, noise and light sensitivity that he had been unable to attend school full time since he hit his head on the side of the pool in September.

The preliminary paperwork for the neuro psych evaluation was comprehensive and there were questions about absolutely every aspect of Sebastian's health and development from birth. *Developmental milestones all normal, except using sign language before he could sit up and reading and writing at age two,* I wrote. *Walked at thirteen months. He took the training wheels off his bike when he was four.* I noted the mild separation anxiety in early childhood, the "I'm Nervous Game", and the anticipational anxiety in middle school.

Socially adept, with excellent choices in friends, athletic and high achieving academically and artistically. Straight A honor student in all honors and AP classes. Water polo and the diving teams in high school. I kept writing.

I was glad I had filled out most of it at home, and grateful my Musikgarten classes were over for the semester. I hoped Sebastian would get some good rest over the holiday and recover. Once my children's choir sang on Christmas Eve, I could relax for a couple of weeks as well.

I just glanced up as Dr. Liu and Sebastian returned to the waiting room for us. Sebastian looked relaxed and comfortable. The two of them joked and made small talk as we turned one corner and then another on the way to Dr. Liu's office. It seemed like a half-mile walk. We went over the details of Sebastian's life and how he got the concussion.

"It was just a two-lap warm-up," Sebastian said, ruefully. "I did a flip turn in the pool and cracked my head on the side of the pool. I misjudged my distance."

"He's competitive," I explained. "He was racing against a swim team kid in the next lane."

Dr. Liu explained that Sebastian would need to have a battery of IQ testing, both verbal and visual-spatial, to see if there had been any brain damage. Sebastian looked drained at the thought. I gave him a sympathetic look as we made the arrangements.

"It was such a pleasure to meet such a nice family," Dr. Liu said as she helped us get our coats.

On the day of the evaluation, Dr. Liu took Sebastian back for his ten-minute check-in, and then we all went back to her office to go over the schedule for the day. The neuro psych evaluation was an entire grueling day of testing, and Sebastian's concussion headache was raging when he emerged at the end of the day. It was a relief he was on winter break.

Christmas came quietly. We kept things simple because of Sebastian's concussion. Eric and I surprised him with a two-week summer course in oil painting at the School of the Art Institute Early College Program in Chicago. Sebastian was thrilled to experience living in the college dorms right in downtown Chicago, and he couldn't wait for June 18th to come.

On December 30, we returned to Dr. Liu to go over the neuro psych evaluation test results. Sebastian had just finished making his coffee at the drinks stand when Dr. Liu walked into the reception area. Dr. Liu's red lipstick was a brighter shade that day, and she looked lovely with her crisp tan slacks, striped blouse, and neat red blazer. She paused in the doorway and looked respectfully at Sebastian. "Congratulations! I've never seen anyone do this before."

Perfect Storm

"This is pretty amazing." Dr. Liu leaned forward on her desk and looked at Sebastian frankly. "I've never seen anyone get a perfect 150 on the verbal portion of the IQ test." She smiled. "Congratulations! This is a first."

"Thanks." Sebastian blushed and fiddled with his sleeve.

"He scored in the very top in third grade when we had to have him tested for the grade promotion. I gave you that report, didn't I?" I looked at Dr. Liu, and then at Eric, who raised an eyebrow.

"Yes." Dr. Liu smiled. "It's just hard to believe." She handed each of us copies of the report. "So, first, Sebastian may have an auditory processing disorder. He noted some difficulties tuning out bothersome noises that should be addressed."

I nodded. Sebastian had mentioned that recently.

"You should take him to an ENT for the preliminary evaluation. Do you have an ENT?"

"I do. I have a great one."

"That's good." Dr. Liu smiled, then glanced back at the reports. "There are also some deficits in the visual-spatial abilities," she continued breezily, "but nothing to be concerned about." She shuffled papers and looked around for something else.

I looked at her and then looked at my copy of the report. I immediately noticed something odd as I studied the chart.

"What's this?" I asked. "Sebastian is borderline impaired on visual-spatial?" I scanned the page anxiously. "That's not just 'some deficits,' that's concerning."

Sebastian sat up next to me and I showed him the report. His forehead wrinkled as he looked at the results. He looked up at Dr. Liu.

"It's just the concussion. Sebastian just needs time," Dr. Liu said smoothly. "He'll be fine."

"Why is there such an enormous gap between his verbal scores and his visual-spatial scores?" I asked. "It makes no sense."

Dr. Liu shrugged.

I sat up straighter and addressed Dr. Liu directly.

"We noticed this gap to a lesser degree when Sebastian had his IQ tested for the grade promotion in third grade. His visual-spatial scores were in the upper average range, which makes no sense for someone as gifted at math as he is." I looked at Eric, who nodded. "I don't understand this. When I asked why there was this discrepancy between his verbal and visual-spatial scores, the psychologist just said that Sebastian quote, unquote, 'isn't as smart as we think he is.'"

Sebastian and I exchanged a look. He rolled his eyes. Dr. Liu sat back and listened.

"As though we pushed for the grade promotion!" I continued, my voice rising slightly. I took a breath and spoke more calmly. "The school came to us. They told us they couldn't meet his educational needs in his current grade. We actually fought the promotion!" I knew I sounded defensive, but everything I told her was true.

I looked at Dr. Liu and simply said, "Genius IQ runs in our family, on both sides."

I looked at Eric, so brilliant, and thought of his father, James, who could make absolutely anything with his hands, despite never having gone to college. An image of one of the quarter-scale model farm implements his dad had engineered and built more than fifty years ago flashed through my mind.

Eric took after his brilliant father in so many ways. He was very grounded in the real, the things and technologies that he could see and touch and understand. His solid reliability and practicality tethered my musical creative brain in a way I appreciated every day.

"We didn't seek out the grade promotion," Eric commented. "We didn't want it, initially."

I shot him a grateful look.

Dr. Liu sat back. "So then why did you choose to do it?"

"It was the least bad option." Sebastian sat up and looked

directly at her. “The other choices sucked.”

I tried to look disapproving, and then laughed.

Eric smiled and agreed. “It was absolutely the least bad of the three choices we got.” He explained about busing Sebastian by himself to the middle school for math and independent study to Dr. Liu.

Dr. Liu nodded. “Schools are great at meeting the needs of average kids.”

I relaxed into my chair slightly and glanced at Eric, who laughed. Sebastian nodded.

“I know.”

I felt some relief at Dr. Liu’s understanding. I gave her a small smile and would have launched into a conversation about how the emphasis on memorization for standardized testing was destroying creativity and real learning, but we had more important things to get to.

“We wanted Sebastian to stay with his friends in third grade, and it was impossible. Anyway, I don’t understand this gigantic gap in his scores. It makes no sense to me.”

“Well, in cases like this, it is possible that Sebastian might have a learning disability called non-verbal learning disability, or NVLD.” Dr. Liu folded her hands and looked at me.

My jaw dropped. “NVLD? I have never heard of that. How could it be possible for a child who is scoring in the ninety-ninth percentile on all standardized tests in both math and language, without any coaching, to have a learning disability?” I looked at Sebastian, who was sitting next to me, just as flummoxed. I turned back to Dr. Liu. “Sebastian is flying through all honors and AP classes. Where is the disability?”

“Well, as I said, it’s just a possibility.” Dr. Liu repeated, waving gently.

“Shouldn’t Sebastian have difficulties with math, with visual-spatial scores this low?” I persisted; my curiosity was piqued. “How do you explain the fact that he’s in honors math and doing the work easily without a tutor, and he’s hardly ever even in class this year because of the concussion? What does this mean? What is NVLD?"

"It's something we sometimes see in kids with this discrepancy, but it's not likely to be an issue in Sebastian's case."

"Not likely to be, or it isn't?"

Dr. Liu shrugged, hands in the air. "Since Sebastian is excelling academically, socially, and physically, then it's unlikely he has a learning disability." She looked slightly exasperated.

"Okay," I sat back, mollified, but still filled with questions. "But he's clearly impaired since the concussion. His visual-spatial scores previously were in the upper average range in third grade. Now he's borderline impaired. Is this deficit going to be permanent?" I looked anxiously at Sebastian and back at Dr. Liu.

Dr. Liu put her elbows on her desk and smiled reassuringly. "Oh, no. There is nothing to worry about." She looked at Sebastian. Their eyes met, and Dr. Liu's voice became more confident. She was back on firm ground now. "You just need more rest, and in a month or two, everything will be okay. You just need more time to heal." She smiled and turned back to me. "There is no reason to believe there is any permanent brain damage from the concussion."

Sebastian and I both sagged back in our chairs when we heard the good news. Eric reached over and squeezed my hand, and Sebastian looked me in the eyes with relief. I reached over and gave his hand a squeeze, too.

Dr. Liu changed the subject. "Sebastian does have some anxiety related to all the missed schoolwork."

I nodded. It was true.

"It would be best to start some therapy."

"Can I do therapy with you?" Sebastian asked, his face open and hopeful.

I wondered what Sebastian saw in her, as I didn't find this doctor terribly helpful. Despite that, Sebastian obviously had formed an attachment in his short time with her. Dr. Liu explained that she didn't offer private therapy, and Sebastian concealed his disappointment. I had several friends who were therapists, so I said I would ask around and find a good one. After friendly goodbyes we headed home.

"After such a crummy year, we deserve some fun. We should plan a trip for this summer," I suggested in the car on the way home. "What was your favorite vacation?"

"Colorado," Eric said. "Snowmobiling in the mountains." He paused, reflecting. "And the snow tubing was pretty awesome."

"That was fantastic, wasn't it." I smiled at Eric then, and he squeezed my hand and gave me a little smile back.

"What was your favorite trip?" Eric asked.

"My favorite memory is hard to pick," I said, considering. I have so many memories. "I think my favorite was going skiing at Chestnut Mountain." I shot a smile over my shoulder to Sebastian.

He glanced up and grinned back. "We had thirteen runs in a row without falling getting off the ski lift!"

A day or two later Sebastian told me he was having trouble remembering things.

"I have this really clear memory of this time in first grade, and then I really can't remember anything until middle school." His face was distraught.

My eyes widened and I could feel my heart rate climbing as I stood. I tried to speak, and nothing came out. I turned around again all the way to face him.

"Are you serious?"

"Yeah."

I glanced at the clock on the microwave. It was after six. At nine the next morning I called Dr. Liu and scheduled an appointment for January 5.

***

"Want a check-in, bud?" Dr. Liu was crisp and ironed as usual, and her pink striped Oxford shirt matched her lipstick.

I read the news. When they returned ten minutes later to retrieve me, Sebastian looked much more relaxed. We sat together, and Dr. Liu casually explained that she was not at all concerned about Sebastian's memory issues.

"It's just the concussion," she assured us, "combined with some anxiety."

Sebastian and I exchanged a glance.

"He is anxious, that's for sure," I agreed. But I'd never heard of anxiety causing memory problems. I felt suspicious and not terribly reassured. "He's missed so much school since September. I know it's been stressful for him. He is a perfectionist, we know that."

"You have a 504 plan set up, right?"

"Yes, we've had one since October. The school has been great. They've reduced so many of the expectations," I said. Then I looked at Sebastian's stressed-out face. "You have always been so hard on yourself."

"I want to do well, and I've missed a lot, that's all." He crossed his arms.

"Kids often get anxious in situations like this. The high-achieving ones," Dr. Liu said, with a sympathetic nod at Sebastian. "They have a tougher time with missing so much school. You've got a really responsible son." Dr. Liu smiled at Sebastian. "Many times, I have seen patients improve their memory when they go on medication."

I was doubtful, to be honest. Dr. Liu seemed like she didn't really know the answer, and so prescribing a pill was all she had in her arsenal. *However*, I thought, *Sebastian does have anxiety from missing so much school.* I had resisted medicating his anxiety before now out of concern for what long-term effects psychotropic medications might have on his developing brain. Now that he was getting older, I thought maybe it might not be a bad idea. His anxiety was abnormally high given the reality of our peaceful and pretty ordinary life.

I asked Dr. Liu for a recommendation for a child psychiatrist, but she didn't have one. She suggested we see our family doctor instead. I trusted Dr. Fredericks, so I nodded. Dr. Liu explained that Sebastian should postpone beginning driver's ed until the summer. She said his reaction times would be slower until the concussion fully healed.

"That's fine with me," Sebastian agreed reasonably. "I can barely keep up with what I've got."

When we got home, I emailed Sebastian's school counselor asking him to drop the driver's ed class, and then I made an appointment with Dr. Fredericks for Sebastian's anxiety for January 10. My Musikgarten classes restarted the next week and I spent the evening sorting all my registrations and going over the music for my church choir. It was Epiphany, and my Cherubim choir children were singing "This Little Light of Mine." I reviewed the choreography and went through the spring musical music.

***

"I don't feel comfortable prescribing anti-anxiety medications to children." Dr. Fredericks's voice was genuinely concerned but regretful. Her thick brown waves were now liberally streaked with silver and swept up into a neat bun. Her natural beauty was accentuated with laugh lines and some peach-colored lip gloss that matched her blouse beneath her white doctor's coat.

I respected her honesty and appreciated how seriously she considered our concerns. She recommended we see her personal friend, the child psychiatrist Dr. Gina Marshall. Dr. Fredericks said she "trusted Dr. Marshall completely." We left satisfied, and at home I called and scheduled an appointment with Dr. Gina X. Marshall for the eighteenth of January.

Dr. Marshall's office was quite far from us in Shorewood. We had an hour-long session, Sebastian and I together. Dr. Marshall seemed nice and prescribed Lexapro for Sebastian's anxiety. Sebastian and I were both relieved to have taken this step, and we were hopeful Sebastian would experience some relief from his anxiety soon.

I picked up the prescription that night. Sebastian took one dose of Lexapro the next day and a second one on the morning of the twentieth of January. Donald Trump's inauguration day was chaotic with protests and heavy news coverage. When I picked up Sebastian from school that day, he said he didn't feel well. As we drove out of the parking lot, his shoulder suddenly spasmed and froze, right up by his ear.

As we drove home, different muscles froze and then relaxed. His leg suddenly extended out and froze, straight out. When we got home, Sebastian couldn't straighten his leg at all as he staggered into the house. I immediately checked the warning for Lexapro that came from the pharmacy. It said to call the doctor immediately, and that muscle spasms could be a sign of something called serotonin syndrome. The information indicated that serotonin syndrome was very serious and could be life-threatening.

Sebastian and I both have drug allergies, so I take all drug reactions seriously. I am cautious, but not hysterical, so I first called Dr. Marshall's office and left a message with the answering service. With our past drug reactions, either our prescribing doctors or the doctor on call had always returned our call regarding drug reactions in ten minutes or under. This time, I waited twenty minutes without a response, and then I called again. Sebastian's muscle spasms worsened as we waited. We waited ten more minutes without a response, and then I called 911.

The paramedics bundled Sebastian onto the gurney and gave him an IV, while Sebastian's legs and arms took on a life of their own. Without volition, his limbs cramped and spasmed so badly that his legs would rise up off the bed, his feet and arms twisting in stiff, weird, and unnatural ways.

"I've never seen a reaction like this before," the treating physician at the ER said. "I'm going to call Dr. Marshall's office. She is the prescribing physician."

The ER doctor ducked out to make the phone call and Sebastian arced backwards in the bed; his entire body froze like an ancient victim of the volcanic eruption of Mt. Vesuvius at Pompeii.

"Can you breathe?" I cried, holding his stone arm. "Can you breathe?"

Sebastian lay, back arched on the bed, stiff and unmoving. He strained against the invisible bonds, fighting for air. The seconds ticked by in slow motion, and then suddenly, whoosh, he gasped for air as though released from a giant's grip.

The ER doctor walked in and his stressed eyes met mine. I looked at the doctor's anxious face, feeling my own panic rising. Sebastian's hand was in mine, now made of flesh and bone again, and I couldn't let go. The doctor's face was stiff and tight, and he bit off his words as he spoke.

"I couldn't reach the prescribing physician, so I am going to call poison control."

Purple Face

I gasped, and the ER doctor spun on his heels and disappeared out the door. I held Sebastian's hand tightly, and moments later, the asphyxiating muscle spasm crushed down on his body again. I couldn't take my eyes off his panicking face as his back arched uncontrollably, his neck tendons like cords.

"Can you breathe?" I cried, afraid to take my eyes off him. "Can you breathe?"

Iron bands surrounded his chest as he fought for air. Seconds ticked by like hours. Just when I thought alarms would sound, he gasped hugely, inhaling as though surfacing from a deep dive. Again and again Sebastian succumbed to the muscular spasms.

He was released hours later with no medication or instructions other than to stop taking the Lexapro and to return to the ER if the symptoms worsened. For at least a week afterwards, Sebastian continued to have major muscle spasms that temporarily stopped his breathing.

***

"It's not your fault," I said, and it was true.

Dr. Fredericks relaxed, her worried eyes magnified behind the gold-framed glasses. She had been so surprised and apologetic at Sebastian's follow-up appointment that I could not blame her. It was not her fault that Dr. Marshall or her staff failed to respond to Sebastian's emergency room visit. With more than twenty years of pleasant history with Dr. Fredericks, I couldn't be angry with her for another doctor's failure. I regretfully told Dr. Fredericks that we would not be returning to see Dr. Marshall, and she said she understood.

Sebastian spasmed so badly he stopped breathing twice during this appointment.

***

"Dr. Sheltze is very, very precise." Dr. Andrei Bucholz crossed his slim legs and smiled reassuringly over his reading glasses.

Sebastian's new psychologist was charming. He was a little short, friendly and warm, with a cap of curly red hair that kinked in little ringlets in a halo around his face. I was there for this first intake appointment without Sebastian present. Dr. Bucholz was appropriately appalled when I told him that the ER doctor had needed to call Poison Control. I appreciated Dr. Bucholz's facial expression as I shared that news.

"Thank you so much." I exhaled with relief. "We need a better child psychiatrist, one that will return phone calls in an emergency. Dr. Sheltze sounds perfect." The tension in my face and shoulders left me and I gestured at the paintings on the walls. "These paintings are lovely. Did you paint them?"

"No, they are from my patients." Dr. Bucholz flashed his dimpled smile, his freckles splashed across his face in a way that made him look younger than the mid-sixties I guessed he was. "My bachelor's degree was in art therapy. You should tell Sebastian to bring his paints and brushes when he comes."

At dinner I filled everyone in, and Sebastian brightened up considerably at the news that Dr. Bucholz was an art therapist.

"I'm glad he had a recommendation for a child psychiatrist," Eric said. "It sounds like a good fit."

At the table I asked Sebastian how his memory was. We decided to look at old photos after dinner to try to jog some memories. Eric was watching one of his TV shows, *Oak Island* or *Gold Rush*, and he had obligingly put on his noise-canceling headphones. He knew he'd have to listen to me complain about the total absence of plot and the annoyingly dramatic canned crescendos that cycled over and over. He had purchased the headphones back when Sebastian was in preschool.

I had started singing again when Sebastian was three, and I had a little time to myself with him at preschool. My big soprano voice had matured into a cathedral-sized Wagnerian that blasted through our modest house like an air horn in an elevator. Eric bought the headphones in self-defense, and I appreciated them when he watched his dirt shows. It was a win-win purchase.

Now, sitting on the sofa with Sebastian by my side, I opened the computer and looked at the pictures of Sebastian as a baby. It had been a while since I had seen his baby book. I felt a rush of nostalgia and tenderness as I remembered how small he was. At seven and a half pounds, he was perfectly average in both height and weight, but still so little. A picture of his first bath popped up and I grinned; the blue of the plastic baby tub matched Sebastian's eyes as they looked directly into the camera, his fuzz of blond hair spun gold in the light from the kitchen window.

"When was the last time we looked at these pictures?" I wondered. "It's been years."

"I don't know, Mom," Sebastian shrugged, looking at his phone.

"I think it was when you were three and you thought you were adopted," I explained.

"I thought I was adopted?"

"You saw something about adoption on *Sesame Street* or something, and I had to pull out your baby book to show you that you were really mine." I looked at him, smiling, and he raised an eyebrow.

"Bummer."

I cracked up, and we looked at a few baby pictures, with me telling him all about who gave him each toy or outfit, and whose arms he was lying in. In the pictures he gazed peacefully up at every face. We moved onto the toddler photos next, and then the preschool ones. Each picture cuter than the next, I talked about each memory of Sebastian; where we were, who we were with.

I clicked the scroll to see what was on the next page, and a gorgeous photo of Sebastian popped up. In that photo, three-year-old Sebastian sat laughing at a table. His eyes were aglow from the flash and from pure joy. His little hand reached out, starfish-like, and his eyes looked straight into the camera, blue and intense. I smiled and turned to Sebastian.

"Oh, look!" I cried, delighted. "Who's that?"

Sebastian looked at the photo. He stared a moment, irritated, and then he shrugged. "How would I know?"

I blinked and froze, then looked back at the photo, so obviously Sebastian. Then I turned slightly and looked at him. He glanced at me, and then turned back to the photo, annoyed.

"You don't know who that is?" I pointed at the picture of him.

"I have no idea."

"Are you serious?" I couldn't take my eyes off him.

Sebastian scowled, upset that he didn't know the correct answer. Sebastian always knew the right answer to every question on every test. The concussion had set him back with headaches and exhaustion, but he was still the same brilliant person I had always known. I could count on one hand the number of times I'd had to help him with homework, and then only briefly. He bent in to take a closer look at the photo of his own face. I watched him, concerned.

"How should I know?" He shrugged and pulled away.

I gaped at him.

Sebastian glanced at me, and then tried again. This time he intently scrutinized the photo. He was visibly frustrated, his jaw tight. It was obvious that he genuinely had absolutely no idea who this stranger in the photo was. I felt my breath go out of me.

"Are you kidding me?" I asked, even though I could see that he was dead serious. "That's you." I pointed at his little toddler face in the photo.

Sebastian looked again, carefully. "Okay," he agreed, unconvinced.

Completely stunned, I felt like I was moving in slow motion. I pointed to another face in an adjacent photo. It was Eric, fifteen years younger, but obviously him. "Who's this?"

Sebastian took a long, hard look and considered.

"I'm not sure,' he said thoughtfully. "Is it Dad, maybe?"

He was obviously guessing, not certain. The laptop slid off my lap. I could hardly breathe. I pulled the laptop back and quizzed Sebastian. Me, Eric, Eric's brother David, David's wife

Kathy: Sebastian was guessing, but not knowing. My mind raced furiously. How could he not recognize his own face, or our faces?

"Eric!" I reached across Sebastian and shook Eric's arm. "Eric!"

Eric looked at me, surprised, and took his headphones off. I explained what I'd just seen happen and suddenly I had a memory. I told them about the time when Sebastian colored Snow White solid purple from the waist up. He was two and a half, and he used to love coloring Snow White so much that I frequently had to buy him new packs of markers just to replace the worn-out yellow one.

"You know, I think Sebastian's had this problem recognizing faces all his life! As I looked over your artwork," I said to Sebastian, "I saw that you had neatly and precisely colored the top half of Snow White solid purple from the waist up. It was weird, because you were two and a half, and you were not scribbling."

"What happened?" Sebastian asked. "What did you do?"

"I remember saying as I passed by, "That's cute! You put Tinky-Winky in a Snow White skirt.' You used to love the Teletubbies when you were a baby, and you had all the dolls."

Sebastian rolled his eyes.

"You had the NuuNuu vacuum, too," Eric laughed. "When you pulled the Tubby Toast on a string, the NuuNuu vacuumed it up its nose."

Sebastian flushed. "Dad."

"You used to laugh hysterically when I pulled that string and put it on your tummy when you were a baby," I added.

"Stop. You are both so embarrassing."

Sitting there on the sofa with my teenage son beside me, I could picture Sebastian at the table with his Tubbies all around him, keeping him company as he colored.

"You know, I used to think you kept your toys around you as you colored for company. Only child, you know? But I think you were using them as a visual reference."

"I do use visual references for my art." Sebastian looked

thoughtful.

As I reflected on this old memory, suddenly I remembered the odd sensation of something being awry as I looked more closely at his coloring page.

"You know what? I remember feeling almost a disorientation, a weirdness, when I saw what you had done. You had colored Snow White solid purple, from the waist up. Her face was completely purple, and neither Tinky-Winky nor Snow White has a purple face!"

Eric looked at me, eyebrow cocked.

"Don't you understand?" I continued. "Sebastian was coloring every part of the figure in the lines, exactly correctly, except for the face."

Eric nodded, thoughtful.

At that exact moment, sitting on the sofa beside Sebastian, I knew without a doubt Sebastian had something wrong with his ability to recognize faces. My child, who at the age of fifteen drew faces with almost photographic realism, couldn't recognize his, or anyone else's, face. I knew this fact with absolute certainty, but I had no idea how it was possible. I felt struck by lightning, struck dumb.

I knew something else, too, with the same certainty. This problem was not from the concussion. He had had this difficulty for a long time, I knew, but I wondered if it was possible he could have been born this way. Sebastian had had zero trauma or serious illness. He'd never been left alone with a babysitter while awake before the age of three. Sebastian's purple face coloring happened before the age of three. It could not have been a babysitter; I knew that for a fact.

We talked about my memories of that time. I remembered thinking Sebastian had been trying to create a picture of Snow White wearing a purple Teletubby suit, so I showed him how to color all around the edges of her face in purple to make the little Teletubby hood. I had felt so odd about Sebastian's purple face coloring that I considered bringing him to Dr. Fredericks over it. I knew I had made a conscious decision to watch and see what would happen.

"I thought that if it continued," I said, "I would take you to the doctor, but you only did it for about a week, and never again. That was the one and only time that I ever saw you fail to differentiate faces."

"So, you didn't take me to the doctor?" Sebastian asked.

"No. You started coloring all the faces just as accurately as you did everything else after that week. Once I pointed out how to draw the Teletubby hood around Snow White's face, you must have realized you had made a mistake by coloring the skin purple. You corrected your own error." I had another realization. "You had all normal developmental milestones. I was pretty sure of the reaction I would get if I took in my perfectly healthy, brilliant two-year-old who'd had all normal developmental milestones and said, 'Sebastian colored Snow White's face purple. I think there's something wrong.'"

Eric circled his finger by his temple. "Cuckoo."

We talked about how Sebastian was coloring all the Disney character faces perfectly accurately before he went to preschool, in the lines. That was just weeks after the purple face coloring incident.

"I vividly remember you blotting your red marker tip on your index finger next. You used to press your red-stained finger onto her cheeks to make a gentle blush, no hard edges. You were three. When I asked you how you knew to do that, you told me your babysitter taught you."

Sebastian sat back and nodded thoughtfully.

"Well, I do use visual references in my artwork, but most artists do. There's nothing odd about that."

"How do you recognize me?" I asked. "I know you recognize me."

"Everything has characteristics."

"What are my characteristics?"

"You are tall/blonde/glasses."

That night I made it my mission to figure out what was happening. I was up until three in the morning before I found my answer. I'm not ashamed, I used Dr. Google. I Googled everything I could think of.

Googling "facial recognition" brought up lots of interesting things about facial recognition technology, but nothing useful. Finally, I Googled "visual-spatial memory and facial recognition problems." Bonanza! Eagerly I read.

The inability to recognize things was a neurological problem called agnosia, and I learned there were several different types. According to Dr. Google, there was something called prosopagnosia, or face blindness, and it was very, very rare. I struggled over how to pronounce it. I sounded it out. Pro-soap-ag-nosia? I shrugged. It would have to do.

According to Dr. Google, people who are face-blind often use physical characteristics to identify others, rather than facial features. That makes sense, I thought. Tall/blonde/glasses. I am tall/blonde/glasses.

Wonder filled me as I considered all this information. There were different types of agnosias, too, I learned. There was an object agnosia, I read, where people couldn't recognize objects, and an environmental agnosia. I tried and failed to imagine what it must be like to not recognize your environment. *How scary,* I thought, and I kept reading.

As I read, I discovered that there was a finger agnosia as well. The article explained that people with finger agnosia couldn't recognize their, or others', fingers. *Thank goodness Sebastian doesn't have that,* I thought to myself. *He could never do his art if he couldn't recognize his own fingers.* I kept reading, so fascinated I couldn't tear my eyes away.

My mind was buzzing when I finally got into bed at three in the morning. I punched Big Squishy down and shook Eric's shoulder.

"Wake up!" I hissed. Eric was buried under the down comforter, fast asleep. He grunted. "I figured it out! I know what it is."

"Hmmm?"

I shook his shoulder. "Wake up! I know what's wrong with

Sebastian."

Eric looked blearily at me and closed his eyes again. "Okay."

"It's called prosopagnosia!" I said, so relieved to share the news. "It's a real thing. It's called 'face blindness.'"

Eric opened his eyes again and blinked at me. "Okay." He started to roll back over.

"Wait! There's this other kind. This finger agnosia thing," I continued. "Who knew that there's a switch in your brain for recognizing fingers?" I lay on my back looking up at the dark ceiling in wonder.

"M'kay," he said groggily, and rolled over.

"Just imagine," I said, wide awake. "It's amazing! Flip the light switch: fingers on, fingers off."

"Ummhmm." Eric pulled the covers up and went back to sleep.

I lay in the dark room, imagining fingers on/fingers off. Faces on/faces off.

Fruit and Fiber

First thing in the morning I called Dr. Liu's office and explained that Sebastian had prosopagnosia, and that he couldn't recognize his own face or anyone else's in the photos we were looking at. I asked for the first available appointment. They booked us for February 3.

The rest of the day was a whirlwind of cleaning, teaching, and errands.

I barely had time to catch my breath after putting tacos on the table. It was Tuesday, and Sebastian had group at church that night.

As he stuffed his feet into his black high-top Converse, he said, "I'm glad I'm not taking driver's ed this semester."

"Me, too," I replied as I grabbed my car keys from the hanger over the kitchen desk. "I'm glad Dr. Liu suggested it. Your reaction times are definitely impaired."

"My concentration is terrible too." Sebastian grabbed his jacket.

"Come on. Let's go. We're late."

'I'm coming." He had one arm in the sleeve of his winter coat when he said, "Is driver's ed where they teach all the names of the streets and stuff?" He stuck his other arm into his coat sleeve and zipped up.

I shoved my right foot into my winter boot as I threw on my winter jacket. We were late again. Tuesdays were so busy. "I guess. Sort of. You just kind of figure it out as you become a more experienced driver. Why?"

"I feel like I don't know where all the streets go." Sebastian bumped his hip against the new dryer as he headed out to the garage. "Ouch." He closed the garage door. "Like how to get to group."

"You just don't pay attention because you aren't driving. I don't pay any attention to where we are going when your dad is driving." I grabbed my purse and stepped out into the messy garage. "Once you start driver's ed, you'll figure it out fast."

"Are you sure?" Sebastian asked, as we got in the car and buckled up. "Like, the compass directions and everything?"

We are going to be really late, I thought. I put the car in drive and headed down our street, hoping I hit all the lights just right. *This is the third time we've been late.* I sighed.

"Sure," I said. "Let's practice. We are headed north on First Street and we're crossing Main." *Got one green,* I thought to myself, as we cruised through the intersection. *Maybe we'll make it after all.* "When we turn right at this stop sign up here, that's Gerald Drive." I glanced at Sebastian. He was listening carefully. "What direction are we going when we turn right?"

He thought for a moment. "East."

"Yup. Then at the light we go left on Jackson." My heart leapt as the left turn arrow turned green just as we pulled up. I breathed a sigh of relief. "Now what direction are we going?"

"North again."

I quizzed him on the street names and the compass directions all the way. At nine o'clock, I picked up Sebastian from the church. On our way home, I quizzed him backwards on the names of the streets and the compass directions. He got every answer right. We were just taking off our coats when I said, "It gets easier when you are driving all the time. It just comes with practice."

I can still see Sebastian's face as he fell on the kitchen floor. He was in an agony of frustration and despair. He was shaking and rocking and sobbing as he covered his face with both hands. Frightened, I dropped my coat and scarf on the kitchen floor and then knelt down beside him. I put my hand on his back and touched his arm.

"What's the matter?" I asked, my heart rate rising. "What's wrong?"

I searched his face, trying to understand what had just happened. I had never seen him like this in my entire life. He was having a complete panic attack, sobbing and shaking, and I didn't know why or what to do. I stared at him.

"What's going on? Tell me what's the matter!" I could feel his rib cage shaking through his down winter coat as he gasped and cried in despair.

"I just don't get it! I just don't understand where everything is."

I stared at him again, breathless. I choked, and then finally managed to say, "What do you mean, you don't understand where everything is?" I was incredulous. "You just got every answer right." I searched his face, trying to understand, and I held his shoulders as he gasped. "You knew the compass directions and the street names."

"Those street names are just words, Mom!" he burst out, angrily. "They don't *MEAN* anything!"

I pulled back and just stared at Sebastian. I had never seen him more serious about something in my life. *What the fuck?* I thought. I pulled away and sat back, watching him intently, his agonized eyes begging me to understand.

Quietly I asked him, "What do you mean, 'they are just words?'" I couldn't take my eyes off him.

Instead of answering, Sebastian leapt up and ripped a sheet of notebook paper from the spiral notebook on the counter. He grabbed a pen from the desk and wrote the street names on the left side:

First Street

Main

Gerald

Jackson

Elm

Maple

Sebastian drew a bubble cloud around the words, and on the right side of the paper he wrote a single word: Streets. He bubbled the word streets in a separate bubble, far to the right side of the paper. I watched him with a mix of fascination and horror. What was he trying to tell me? I had no idea, until suddenly he drew a "does not equal" sign in the middle.

He looked at me intently, willing me to understand him, and then said slowly and definitely, "The street names are just words.

I don't know where they are. There is no connection between the names and the places."

Sebastian spoke those words with as much conviction as I have ever heard any human ever say anything. His eyes pleaded with mine for understanding, and I stared into his eyes uncomprehendingly.

"I don't know where Main Street is," he burst out.

The floor dropped out from under me. *Oh, my God,* I thought. *How is that possible?* Every hair on my arms stood up.

Slowly, I replied, "How can you not know where Main Street is?" Sebastian's eyes were locked on mine, serious and uncompromising. The hairs on my head rippled upwards like a wave of frigid water and I gasped, "We drive on it every day. It is two blocks from our house! How could you not know where it is?"

Sebastian hid his agonized face behind his arms and rocked, sobbing on the kitchen floor.

I struggled to breathe, wondering what on earth was wrong with him. I reached for him. His face was contorted in fury, fear, and frustration. I stared at him, unsure if he wanted my touch or not, so I just stood there, gaping. My brilliant child, who knew more about just about everything than I did, didn't know where he lived. It was impossible.

"I don't know!" he cried "I don't know where any of them are."

Something in my brain clicked; not recognizing faces, not recognizing places. A puzzle piece from the reading the night before clicked. "Face blindness and environmental blindness often occur together." Sebastian had environmental agnosia, too! Right then, I knew it.

My son was lost. I stared at him, curled on the floor, his face wracked with pain. I rocketed from incredulity to terror. If he couldn't recognize his own environment, how could I explain where Main Street was to him? Images swirled through my mind: Sebastian riding his bike; walking to school; running through the back yard; turning cartwheels on the lawn. I could see him ice skating and doing clumsy twirls on his very first trip to the ice rink when he was four.

My son didn't know where he lived. I felt my hair stand up in that old familiar feeling, ten inches tall. The world tipped and whirled around, beneath me. He was lost. I had to help him to understand. I had to show him where he lived.

And then I saw it. If he couldn't recognize the roads with vision, maybe he could feel them, like Helen Keller with the water in *The Miracle Worker*. I saw the bowl of apples on the kitchen table. I reached out and grabbed one and thunked it on the table.

"This is our house." I said. "And I don't know how many other houses are on our block."

"Seven."

His voice was sure. He'd counted. He knew. I looked at him, and he stood up beside me and pulled out seven more apples, one at a time, and lined them up to the left of our apple. I looked wildly around the room and spotted a skein of red yarn on the counter. I grabbed a pair of scissors. I snipped a tiny piece of yarn and lay it on the table, so it came out from our apple "house."

"This is our driveway."

Sebastian, face intent, watched my every move. I cut a long piece of yarn and connected it to our yarn driveway, making a large circle on the table.

"This is our street, Cortway."

Sebastian's eyes followed as I lay the yarn down. His entire being focused on that piece of red string. I cut another shorter piece of yarn.

"This is Glenview." I bisected the circle, laying the Glenview Road piece behind our row of apple houses and across the Cortway circle. Sebastian shifted his weight, and stared hard at the table, not comprehending.

First Street was a busier road, so I grabbed my scarf from the floor and laid it across the left side of Glenview.

"First Street."

Main was a busy four-lane road. I grabbed Sebastian's scarf and stretched out on the table closest to us, parallel to our row of apple houses, and intersecting my First Street scarf on the left side.

"This is Main."

I looked at the mess of yarn and apples and scarves strewn across our kitchen table. Sebastian was standing beside me, staring, willing himself to understand but obviously not. His eyes searched for meaning, intent and focused, but no understanding came.

"Touch it," I said.

He glanced at me, hesitant.

"You can't just look at it. You have to touch it."

Slowly, Sebastian reached out his hand. His hand went directly to our apple house on the right side of the line of apples.

"That's our house," I said. Sebastian glanced at me and pulled his hand away from the apple.

"Touch it." I insisted. "You can't just look. You have to touch it."

Carefully, almost fearfully, Sebastian reached out and touched the apple again. I put my hand over my mouth and watched in silence as he drew his index finger down the side of the apple and lightly landed on our snippet of yarn driveway.

"That's our driveway," I whispered through my fingers.

Time slowed, and there was nothing in the universe except my son and this cartography of fruit and fiber. Sebastian was concentrating like I have never seen him concentrate. His entire being was focused on the mystery beneath his hand. His finger lightly landed on our street.

"That's our street." I could barely breathe. "Go left."

I held my breath as he traced the red yarn up and around to where it intersected with the Glenview strand.

"That's Glenview." I whispered. "Go left."

Sebastian traced the red yarn to the left and touched my plum-colored scarf.

"First Street." I could barely whisper. "Come towards you."

The concentration on Sebastian's face was intense and fixed, his eyes determined to find meaning.

He traced my scarf along the table towards him. His index finger touched his gray scarf, running east-west across the table. I breathed. "Main Street."

Sebastian's brilliant blue eyes widened, his mouth opened, and comprehension bloomed across his stunning face. He turned, and those unknowable, fathomless eyes met mine and I saw my child for the very first time. He nodded.

I felt faint. I grabbed the back of the kitchen chair to steady myself. My heart raced. My brilliant, genius child understood where the main road by his house was for the very first time. His eyes lifted to mine, and we looked at each other, not breathing.

In a split second, everything made sense. The separation anxiety, the crying at drop off for three years, the "I'm Nervous Game," the fear of getting lost when he went to middle school. The pieces of the puzzle came tumbling together.

I stood there, memories pouring over and through me. I could hear the sound of Sebastian's soprano child voice singing "I took off my training wheels, so appa dacka shpayniels." I could feel his little toddler body clinging to me, his wet face against my neck as he held on, crying at preschool drop-off, "When can I take Algebra!" I saw him catching a pass at water polo and scoring his first goal. I saw his back as he rode down the street on his bike with April to the park. I could see him chopping carrots and flipping cartwheels, and I heard the thwop of his badminton racquet as he lobbed the birdie over the net to me. I saw him hitting a homerun and chasing the soccer ball down the field and sinking his first goal. I saw him drawing a face, the eye perfect and almost lifelike in its realism. I felt his small body in my arms, the sweet tug of his arms around my neck as I stood in the grocery store, me feeling simultaneous concern, confusion, and even irritation. "I'm nervous, Mama," he said. "I'm nervous."

Amazing Grace, how sweet the sound. My seeing child is blind. My blind child can see. I had no idea how this could be possible, but I knew that it was true. Sebastian was blind. Sebastian could see. He was a miracle. I was a monster. I didn't know. I didn't see.

He was right in front of our eyes, and nobody knew. Nobody saw. Nobody warned me. Nobody noticed.

"Oh, my God. Oh, my God," I cried. "I'm so sorry. I am so sorry." I turned and hugged him, and he was holding me back, his tall, slender frame so familiar in my arms. We fell to our knees on the kitchen floor, not letting go. "I'm so sorry, baby. I'm so sorry." I sobbed. "I didn't know."

"What, Mom?" he asked, his face devastated. "What's the matter?"

"I am so sorry, baby."

"What's the matter? Why are you crying?"

I took his face in my hands, the prickle of his short hair at the nape of his neck braille against my fingers as I read my son for the very first time. I stared into his eyes.

"You're blind, honey." I cried, tears running down my face. Sebastian gaped at me, not comprehending.

I took a breath and tried to steady my voice. I was shaking and I could feel my hands tremble as I reached to hold both of his hands. I looked into his limpid and incomprehensible gaze, the sky of his amaurotic reality blue and depthless. His eyes searched mine. Blind eyes on blind eyes, we stared at each other in ontological horror.

Understanding cracked the porcelain veneer of his china-blue perfection. Sebastian's twin circumpunctual mysteries contracted like black holes, and then exploded with shock and recognition. Monster and miracle, we stared at each other in grief and horror. He inhaled sharply, almost bending double as if punched. I ducked down and caught him in my arms.

"Oh, sweetheart. I am so sorry. I am so, so sorry."

Our tears blurred into one river as Sebastian's long arms wrapped my shoulders, his cheek against mine. His chest and shoulders shook as we knelt together on the kitchen floor, a monster of obliviousness and a miracle of oblivion; yin and yang.

"You don't look blind," I cried. "I didn't know."

King of the Hill

"Eric!" I shouted. "Eric!" He was sitting on the couch with his back to us, not six feet away, but he was wearing his noise-canceling headphones and watching his dirt show.

"Dad!" shouted Sebastian, as I got to my feet and walked around the couch, waving to get his attention.

"Eric! Take your headphones off!" I shouted urgently, waving in his face.

"Dad!"

"What?" Eric said, his face cross and his brows furled. He pulled off his headphones and looked from my face to Sebastian's. "What's going on?" His eyes softened when he saw our faces. "What happened?"

"Come here!" I said urgently.

"Okay." Cautiously Eric stood and walked around the sofa, stepping over our winter jackets that still lay strewn across the floor. He looked skeptically at the kitchen table with its maze of yarn and scarves and apples. "What's going on?"

"Something just happened," I gabbled, almost incoherent. "I figured it out. I know what's wrong!"

Eric looked at the table, and then at each of us in turn. "Okay?"

I explained everything that had just happened.

"I'm a teacher!" I exclaimed. "I know that look when a kid gets it for the first time. It was unmistakable!"

Eric listened to everything patiently, without comment. He nodded. "Okay?"

I was about to respond, when in my mind's eye, I saw Sebastian taking off on his bike to go to April's house. I gasped, and turned to Sebastian, my mouth hanging open.

"How on earth do you get to April's house?" I asked Sebastian, my eyes wide.

Sebastian slowly seated himself at the kitchen table. His face was thoughtful, pensive. He considered.

"I go this way." He twitched his shoulders in a slight motion to the left. My eyes were glued to him. "And then this way." Left again. "This way." Right, this time. "Then this way." Right again. "Yeah, I think that's right," he said, looking up at me again.

"Oh, my God. Did you just see that?" I asked Eric, desperately, praying for him to see what I just saw, to understand what just happened.

"Yeah," he said, thoughtfully. "That's the way."

"How do you get around the school?" I asked, fascinated. I was pinballing between disbelief, horror, and amazement. *How could this be possible?*

"I count my steps and turns."

Just like that. Like everyone does. Everything I thought I knew exploded all around me. I could not believe what I was hearing from my son. My child. I could not believe what I was seeing, but I knew he was telling the absolute truth. *When you grow up in a house where love is hate and hate is love,* I thought, *it's easier to hold two opposites in your mind at once. Sebastian was blind/not blind.*

"Is that how you get from class to class?" I asked, unable to pull my eyes away.

Sebastian's face was soft, and his eyes were far away, considering.

"I count the hallways and the doorways," he explained. He paused and thought again. "It's harder when I have to go to the computer lab," Sebastian admitted, his face flushing. "I don't know how to get there from the previous class, so I have to go to the regularly scheduled class and then find my way from there." He looked at me, begging me with his eyes to understand.

In my mind's eye, I saw him, three years old at preschool, walking down the hall to the gym, holding his friend's hand. We thought it was so cute. I cried. Tears flowed down my cheeks as I thought of my little child, my son, finding his way through a world he couldn't recognize, without help, his entire life. Devastation and incredulity rocketed back and forth inside me. I looked at him, amazed and also filled with horror and guilt; I felt all three simultaneously.

"Draw me a map." I said, wiping my tears, handing him the spiral notebook and the pen. "Draw me a map of your high school. How do you get to class?" I asked. I watched, terrified of what was coming but desperate to understand. Sebastian took the pen and thought.

"Hmm," he said, considering carefully. "Coming in from the auditorium side." He paused for a moment and thought again. Then he drew a line, in one continuous motion. Without lifting the pen from the paper, a tangled web emerged. There were no halls or classrooms, no gym, no basic map. "There," he said, satisfied. "That's my class schedule."

His pathway through the building was a single tangled line of turns. I looked at Eric, who was quietly standing on the side, observing.

"Do you see that?" I asked him.

"Yeah." Eric nodded, thoughtful but quiet.

Sebastian's face brightened. "You know, I always thought I had really good night vision," Sebastian volunteered. "But now I know I don't use my vision when I move around the house."

My eyes widened. "What do you mean you don't use your vision?" I asked him. "What are you talking about?"

"I never turn the lights on in the evening when you aren't home," Sebastian explained helpfully.

Gravity no longer existed. I felt like I was going to just float off my chair and fly away. Nothing that I knew was real. Nothing real was true.

"I always used to think that I had good night vision, but now I know I'm not using my vision when I walk around at home," he repeated, realizing as he said the words the truth of his experience. "At school I mostly use my vision just to keep from bumping into things. Like our new dryer. That thing gets me every time I pass it," he said with a small laugh. "It's different from the old one and I can't see it."

The new dryer stuck out about six inches further than the old one. I saw Sebastian bump into it on our way out tonight. I glanced at Sebastian's map of his high school, and suddenly I remembered something else. Disbelief filled me. I sat straighter and looked hard at him, hands on hips.

"I helped you study for the geography tests for honors world history freshman year. You sat beside me on the sofa, and I asked you where each city was. The first time you knew almost every answer. You pointed to each one exactly. We practiced twice that week, and then you had them perfectly. You came home from school and told me you were the map games champion. What was that game you played?"

"King of the Hill?"

I inhaled hard and almost shouted. "How did you do that?" There was just so much I couldn't believe. "Can you even picture the boot of Italy?"

"No." He shook his head.

"Then how did you do that?" I persisted, glancing at Eric, who stood impassively watching.

"That was easy." Sebastian smiled. "I just assigned every city a numerical value and plotted them all on an XY axis." He shrugged. "I thought everybody did that."

My jaw dropped. "No. That's not how people do that."

Sebastian's eyebrows lifted in surprise. Then, suddenly, the competitive Sebastian I knew emerged.

His face suffused with pride and he said, "I can do it with the map behind my back." He demonstrated, karate chopping his outstretched left arm, boom. Right there. His face was a warrior's face. "No one can beat me."

I sank back slowly into the chair across from him. Pride filled Sebastian's face; his determination to succeed now written legibly across his expression in a way I could finally read. I felt lightheaded. I looked at Eric, who stood silently observing. I looked back at my son, as fierce and determined as I have ever seen him.

Sebastian is a miracle, I thought to myself. *He is an absolute miracle. My child, who had passed every vision test every year, is blind. He is blind, and yet he sees.*

Grief/pride/fear/wonder/guilt/curiosity/amazement/shock

/sadness. *What is the name of that emotion,* I wondered crazily. Sebastian wasn't blind, I realized. I was. I was blind, but *now* I see. He is blind, *and* he sees.

Right there, right then, in my kitchen, I saw my son for the very first time. My invisible child was suddenly visible. *God help us,* I prayed silently.

At that, I was stunned with grief for all this child had been through. *All those years,* I thought; *all those times that I dropped him off at school.* 180 days in a school year, times two years of preschool. Plus another 180 days of kindergarten. I calculated the horror of the 540 times I unwittingly dropped my blind child off at school, until he finally stopped crying in first grade. I knew he didn't stop being afraid in first grade. He just stopped telling me that his tummy hurt. I felt my head shaking back and forth, and I couldn't collect myself.

Everything made sense now. I felt like our entire world just turned upside down. I abandoned him, over and over again. I left him at school, and he couldn't recognize a single soul. He couldn't find his way. I abandoned my baby. Hundreds of times. The horror of what I did was indescribable. My hands shook and I couldn't breathe.

"Sebastian," I said shakily as I reached out to take his hand in mine. "You can usually tell when someone is blind. It's usually obvious."

Eric nodded.

I glanced at Eric and then continued, "No one ever suggested to us that there was anything wrong with you."

Sebastian looked me in the eye, with those unknowable blue eyes, and I continued. "Not one doctor. No teacher. No friend. No family member." I continued, desperate for him to believe me. "Not one single person ever suggested to us that there was anything wrong with you, ever." *God, please believe me,* I prayed. "We did not know, honey. Oh, my God, we didn't know."

Tears brimmed in Sebastian's eyes. His eyes shimmered, blurred, then cleared when he blinked. His face was drawn as we both stood and reached for one another. He wrapped me in his long arms.

"Not one single person. Ever. Once."

I felt Sebastian's sobs; his ribcage heaved under my arms as he gasped.

"I am so sorry," I cried. "Please forgive me. I'm so sorry. I love you so much."

"I love you, Mom," he said, his voice thick and furred. "You are the best mom in the world."

***

First thing in the morning I called Dr. Liu's office and scheduled an appointment for February 3.

Sebastian's condition was obviously neurological, and my greatest concern was his ability to navigate the wider world. We determined that Sebastian had taught himself three pathways through our tiny neighborhood, his class schedule at his large and extremely architecturally complex high school, and our home. I had no idea if he could ever learn to live independently or how he would be able to work or go to college. I knew we needed immediate assistance getting Sebastian orientation and mobility services.

We marveled at how absolutely Sebastian's vision impairment had been concealed. Being almost six feet tall made me stand out in a crowd for him at pickup time, he told me, and Sebastian was an only child. I was never distracted by other siblings at pickup time, so I knew now that I was always the one recognizing him and finding him in a crowd. Although Sebastian's elementary school was close by, most of his friends were bused in from another town. With the exception of April and the friends on our street, he had been driven to friends' houses all his life. We never saw him get lost.

We talked about Sebastian's oil painting class at the School of the Art Institute in June. The idea of him blindly wandering the Chicago streets terrified me.

Sebastian said firmly, "I want to go. I don't want to cancel.

It's the only good thing I have had to look forward to this year."

"I know, Sebastian. I just don't think it's safe."

"I want to go."

"We have to get you a diagnosis so that you can access orientation and mobility. Let's focus on that first, and then we'll see."

"I want to go."

Sebastian's face was filled with pain. I rubbed his shoulder and looked into his eyes.

"I know. I want you to be able to go. Your appointment with Dr. Liu is on the third. Let's see what she has to say, and what programs there are for people like you. We've got several months to get you ready."

I felt very stressed, because he was a sophomore in high school, and there was so little time left to get help from the school. He should have had orientation and mobility services years ago. Sebastian's oil painting class started on June 18. We didn't have much time and it felt like eons until we saw Dr. Liu again.

***

"Can you recognize your own face?" I asked.

I gathered up the emotion recognition cards I had ordered and looked at Sebastian. He looked straight back at me.

"No," he said flatly. "I can't."

I bought a set of emotion recognition cards because I couldn't stop wondering if I'd been imagining that Sebastian had been responding to my facial expressions all these years. I wondered if I'd been in some major denial. I quizzed him with the emotion recognition cards. Sebastian got them all right but one, and then I made him give the test to me. I missed the exact same card. It was the little girl with her finger pressed to her lips. The answer on the card said "Shy," but Sebastian and I both thought she looked more secretive. She had that glint in her eye.

Sebastian and I talked a lot about what we'd discovered. We

had plenty of time, as he was still doing only half days because of the concussion.

"But your self-portrait! It's gorgeous."

"I use photos for visual reference, Mom. I chart it on a grid. A lot of artists do that."

"But I've watched you draw beautiful, realistic eyes, just sitting at the table. I don't understand."

"Mom, I've drawn so many eyes, it's just muscle memory."

I thought for a moment. "Then, how do you make eye contact with me, if you can't recognize my face?" I asked. It was just so difficult to understand.

He didn't miss a beat. "I look at the point between people's eyebrows," he said, looking straight at me. He looked exactly like he was making eye contact. "Most human beings accept that as eye contact."

I chuckled inwardly. My superhuman baby had been living in a Kryptonite universe with no one the wiser. I inhaled sharply. *Baby pictures!*

"I have baby pictures of you making eye contact from your earliest days!" I stared at him, my eyes on his. "Who taught you to do that?"

He shrugged, blue eyes on my gray. "I don't know. I just do it."

Marble Maze

My Musikgarten classes resumed in a fog. I went through the motions. For the first time I felt disconnected from my families as I tried to piece together the shards of Sebastian's life that I had missed or overlooked. My children's church choir rehearsals were equally distant from my consciousness, as every waking moment I felt consumed by the need to know and understand my son. I missed seeing so much, first from my own protectiveness, but also from the nature of the times we lived in.

Kids played in supervised groups in the suburbs. Sebastian had never been alone in the woods, or even at the mall at the age of fifteen. He and his friends all traveled in packs for safety when they were younger, and then just for the fun of it as they got older. In one moment, we went from being the parents of a gifted kid to parents of a gifted child with a serious disability, and I had no experience with anything like this before.

I had never even heard of agnosia or face blindness before. I alternated wildly between marveling at how extraordinary his accomplishments were with such a severe visual impairment, and terror. Our world was upturned, literally overnight. Everywhere I turned, I saw Sebastian alone, lost, and surrounded by nothing familiar. Suddenly, I was considering a very real future where my son never left my home.

I was consumed with fear about Sebastian's ability to navigate the wider world. I can't explain that terror about his blindness in any other way. The fear a parent has for their child's very survival is a primal one, and the human fear of being blind, I know now, is often more powerful than death. In surveys, parents prefer their child to have a deadly form of cancer over being blind. I was scared to death for him. I'm not ashamed to admit it.

Suddenly, it occurred to me that maybe a guide dog would help him. At least with a dog by his side, Sebastian would not be alone. Drivers would see that he was visually impaired and give him space as he crossed the street. I knew that service dogs reduced anxiety just with their presence, so just having that companionship might help his fear and anxiety.

I called the Seeing Eye guide dog admissions line. The woman who answered the phone listened carefully and asked perceptive questions. She had clearly taken many very emotional phone calls from prospective clients before, and she gave me all her attention. She very kindly and gently explained that a guide dog probably wouldn't likely be much benefit, as Sebastian didn't bump into things. We politely ended the phone call.

I sat on the piano bench and cried.

***

On January 26 I drove to Schaumburg by myself for an intake appointment with the new child psychiatrist, Dr. Norman Sheltze. I arrived at the office ten minutes early and was immediately impressed with the swanky modern decor. It was a very busy practice, with many families in the waiting room, and a huge arrangement of gladiolus and pink Gerbera daisies were artistically arranged in a black vase on the reception desk.

This was an intake appointment without Sebastian present, so I met with a therapist, not the prescribing psychiatrist. We went over everything that had happened, from the concussion to the discovery of Sebastian's visual impairment. I explained how much anxiety Sebastian had experienced over the years as a result of having both face blindness and environmental agnosia and no one knowing. I told her I thought Sebastian probably had PTSD from having gone so long without orientation and mobility training.

The intake person listened carefully, asked lots of questions about Sebastian's development, which was all normal, and was very kind and thorough. She didn't offer any opinions and I didn't have the opportunity to ask her anything, because there was so much to explain. We discussed Sebastian's drug reaction to the Lexapro as well. The hour was over very quickly, as so much had happened. I told her we had scheduled an appointment with Dr.

Sheltze for Wednesday, February 22nd. It felt a long way off.

At home I was tidying up after my Family Music for Toddlers class when the phone rang. It was Lukas Franck, from the guide dog organization, the Seeing Eye. I sat down on the piano bench in surprise and relief. Visions of a heroic German shepherd leading Sebastian around the city danced in my head.

Lukas's pleasant baritone voice was friendly and calm. He asked me how we discovered Sebastian's agnosia, and I explained. I told him about Sebastian taking the training wheels off his bike when he was four, the photos, and everything we had discovered since.

Lukas listened very carefully and then asked many questions about Sebastian's navigation skills. I told him Sebastian had taught himself to count his steps and turns as a toddler, and then I asked if a guide dog would be a possibility for him. Of course, I knew absolutely nothing about guide dogs. Lukas patiently and very kindly explained that the dog did not know the destination; it only helped the person to avoid obstacles.

Lukas went on to carefully explain that the person using the guide dog must be completely in charge of navigating, or else the dog would learn to take advantage. I listened, feeling my hope deflate, but recognizing the logic. Lukas added that the owner also had to completely trust the dog's instincts when it came to avoiding obstacles. He told me that if the person second-guesses the dog's judgment, the dog will lose its training and become a $50,000 pet. Sebastian didn't crash into things, Lukas explained kindly. A guide dog would probably not be a good fit.

A huge wave of sadness passed through me as I listened to the inescapable logic of Lukas's argument. Sebastian would have to learn to travel alone.

"The last thing we would want is to take a dog from someone who needs one more," I said quickly. "Plus, we're allergic to dogs. If we needed a $50,000 allergen, we would rescue one."

Since Nickie and Penny passed away, everyone in the house had been breathing easier. If I hadn't been so upset by all the recent events, I realized, I might have thought of all these things for myself. Fortunately, Lukas had clearly explained this fact, kindly and with great compassion, to many upset parents in the past. I took comfort in the fact that I was obviously not the first with stupid questions, and that he was so compassionate and patient.

Lukas asked to speak with Sebastian, and they had quite a long conversation. I could hear them discussing how Sebastian navigated around the house, the neighborhood, and his school. I was impressed with the genuine concern and compassion I sensed from this kind man. After chatting for about twenty minutes, Sebastian passed the phone back to me.

At the end of the conversation, Lukas made some suggestions and gave me some names and local organizations to contact. There was technology available to help in situations like this. We were not alone. I thanked Lukas for his kindness. His concern and caring lifted my spirit and renewed me. Feeling recharged and comforted, I called the Lighthouse in Chicago and set up an appointment with the technology team. *We can manage this,* I thought. *With the right supports and some technology, Sebastian will be just fine.*

***

"Have you ever heard of something like this?" It was January 31, and I was ugly-crying on the sofa with my dear friend Patty Kelly on the phone. My efforts to be brave had worn off, and the compassion in Patty's voice undid me. With her doctorate in occupational therapy, I had thought that perhaps she could shed some light on Sebastian's vision impairment. It was only minutes into our conversation before I came unglued.

"No," she laughed, kindly, in her special way. "You're the first." Patty paused, considering. "You know, you are really lucky that you discovered this problem before he started driver's ed."

"I know. Can you imagine? I talked about this with Sebastian last night." I swallowed, and choked out, "I told him he really needs to be aware that he may not be able to drive."

"Do you think he won't be able to?"

"I'm not sure." Tears started, again. "He can't navigate at all. When I asked him how he was going to find his way around, he said he plans to just count the intersections as he goes. There could be dozens or hundreds of them! He'll be so distracted counting that I don't think he can focus on what's coming at him."

"Hmmm..."

"I think that maybe with technology he could. Like with a Garmin?" I suggested, hopeful.

Patty told me about a program for visually impaired drivers at a local hospital. She explained they did a very thorough safety assessment before allowing anyone to start the program, and that they had all kinds of technology to help. I wanted to hug her through the phone as I thanked her. She laughed and invited Sebastian and me to the barn to see her mustang, Mini.

I sat back up urgently, remembering Sebastian riding Mini around the ring.

"Did you notice anything at all weird about Sebastian's vision when you met him?" *Maybe I've been in denial,* I thought again, waiting breathlessly for her answer. Patty thought for the briefest moment, and then answered.

"No. Not at all."

I sat back again, relieved. Patty is honest. She would have told me if she saw something. We planned a mini high school reunion for April, chatted a while longer, and then Patty had to go.

"Come see Mini at the barn. Next time you come, we'll hitch her to her cart and you can drive her."

"Are you serious? We would love to." I hung up, relieved and reassured of my sanity, but that feeling didn't last long.

***

"I'll be back at one." The receptionist smiled as she pulled on her jacket. "Do you need anything before I go?"

"Thanks, I'm fine." I replied. I was too anxious to read the news while I waited for Dr. Liu to return from Sebastian's ten-minute check-in. I went over everything that had happened mentally, and my anxiety rose as the minutes passed.

Instead of the expected ten-minute check-in, Dr. Liu kept Sebastian for the entire hour as I fretted anxiously in the waiting room. There was so much I needed to talk to her about, and I truly didn't remember the way to her office through the long maze of passages. I didn't know the office number either. I pictured myself, like a marble in a marble maze, bumping along the walls. With my luck, I'd go the wrong way and miss them, I decided, and we'd be chasing each other around the building. There was no one to ask for directions.

At last I heard their footsteps and voices down the hall. I stood, concerned and upset that I had not been included in this most crucial appointment. It had been an hour, and the appointment time was over. Dr. Liu was walking casually, her arms swinging at her sides, relaxed. She was obviously done.

"That's it then," she said as she waved a dismissive goodbye and turned back the way she came. She had more important work to do, her body language screamed.

Sebastian's face was stricken. I could see that he was upset.

"Wait!" I called as I walked quickly towards her. "Wait! That's it?" I asked, completely shocked. "I need to talk to you! This is really serious."

Dr. Liu swung around and looked surprised at my concern. Reluctantly, she gestured us back towards her office, saying she had a few more minutes.

It was clear that Dr. Liu hadn't believed a single word Sebastian had said. My words came spilling out. The photos, not recognizing his own face, the purple face coloring, the map on the table, the separation anxiety, the "I'm Nervous Game," almost all of it documented in Liu's own report. I showed her the Weschler Intelligence Scale for Children (WISC) scores.

"Look at the gap between the scores." I explained: "The genius-level verbal abilities have masked his visual-spatial deficits. They have given him a false positive in his visual abilities. He's not borderline impaired, he's almost completely impaired."

Dr. Liu frowned doubtfully at me.

"Everything was masked," I explained. "Every clue was disguised as something else. I didn't notice that he couldn't recognize me at pick up," I pressed on, explaining about my height, Sebastian's misdiagnosis in middle school of anticipational anxiety, how he had been driven to his friends' houses all the time.

"We didn't catch the navigation issues because his middle school is so easy to get around," I continued. "It's just a big rectangle, and it's exceptionally well-marked."

I gestured to Sebastian, who was sitting, listening attentively, on my right. "He taught himself his steps and turns in just one trip through his class schedule. It looked like he actually did have anticipational anxiety, because after that one trip through his schedule, his anxiety about getting lost completely disappeared."

Sebastian nodded.

Dr. Liu was listening to me intently, her face concerned, but she did not respond. I had another realization at that moment, and I burst out, "And his high school was so challenging that it took me three days of walking it before I had any idea where *I* was going! It's such a maze, it's notorious. Everyone complains about it. It's an older building that was originally designed as an open-concept school in the seventies, and then was added onto multiple times," I explained. I remembered something. "I actually subbed there once three or four years ago, and I had such a hard time finding my way around that I never went back. I didn't notice that it took Sebastian three days of practice to learn his route there by counting his steps and turns, because it took me just as long with my normal vision."

As I spoke, I saw confusion on Dr. Liu's face. She alternated between belief and disbelief at what I was telling her, and yet I could see she recognized my sincere concern. She looked torn and indecisive for a moment. Suddenly, she made up her mind. Firmly she announced her time was up. She had to go. She had to end the session.

"That's it?" I gasped, incredulous. "But Sebastian needs an Individualized Education Plan at school. He has to have orientation and mobility services! He is going to college in two years and he can't navigate a college campus, or even the mall by himself! We don't even know if he can drive!"

Dr. Liu stood impassively.

"He absolutely has to be assessed at the program for the visually impaired at our local hospital before he can start driver's ed," I said, silently thanking God for Patty's help the other day. "He has only until age twenty-one to access services. I know that services for the visually impaired drop off alarmingly after that. He's got to have a diagnosis for an IEP."

Dr. Liu threw her hands up in exasperation. "I can't help you and I don't know anyone who can," she said firmly. "Good luck with that!"

ACT TWO

Maelstrom Chameleon

"Drawing is the discipline by which I constantly rediscover the world. I have learned that what I have not drawn, I have never really seen, and when I start drawing an ordinary thing, I realize how extraordinary it is, sheer miracle." - Frederick Franck

"They do not see what they look at, hence they know not what they do." - Frederick Franck

It wasn't that my seventeen-year-old, water-polo-playing son's three paintings, two parrots and a post-post neo-expressionist abstract, were hanging in a museum just steps away from Mary Cassatt's *Mother Looking Down, Embracing Both Her Children* that floored me. It was the fact we were still alive at all. It was a year later, December of 2018, and I was staring at a realistic watercolor painting of our green, dusky conure, Mimi. Her black-and-white bird's eye stared impishly back at me from her perch on top of the lid of a Starbucks cold cup, and I couldn't shake the feeling that none of this was real.

I shook my head slightly and glanced around the Albrecht-Kemper Museum of Art, reassured that we were all still there, and then turned my attention back to Sebastian's paintings. In my experience, watercolors were usually misty seascapes of tenuous gray-green swells rolling under tiny sailboats, with tiny rounded v's of gulls in the washed-denim sky above, or else they were garden scenes of lush, vague greenery and flowers. Sebastian's precise feathered exactness of Mimi's multitudinous shades ranging from mid-pickle green to margarita lime surprised my eye, again.

Next to the startling watercolor of Mimi, Kalo the macaw snapped a piece of wood with her nutcracker beak in oil on canvas. I half expected to hear her oddly metallic speech and the crunch of wood as pieces rained down upon the museum floor. Kalo's red-feathered breast contrasted boldly with the creamy white facial skin and black lines around her eyes

I glanced around for Sebastian and didn't see him. Shivers rose up my back, tingling the hairs on the nape of my neck. Lost. I inhaled through my nose and exhaled slowly to calm down. Even this happiest of days was hard to process and enjoy. My knee ached sharply, and I shifted my weight, my feet sore underneath the many extra pounds. In the past year and a half, I had gained back every single pound I'd lost in the eighteen months after my mother died, from the stress of trying to get a diagnosis for Sebastian's visual impairment.

Beneath Mimi and Kalo, two flat, matte-blue headless figures held hands and danced towards me, a third following behind as though trying to catch up. Our family, perhaps, captured on canvas, with what looked to my untrained eye like a joy I recognized but still couldn't allow myself to feel. *I should ask Sebastian,* I thought. *Maybe it isn't us, no matter how much I want it to be.*

I felt envious of the headless people in Sebastian's *Blue Figures* as I shifted my weight again on my arthritic knees and wondered when life would feel real again and if I'd ever lose the weight I'd gained. Without faces, the painted figures didn't have to try to smile, though the love between the painted dancers was obvious to me. I looked to Eric on my right, who was nodding thoughtfully at Sebastian's work. He caught my glance and quirked his lip at me.

"Pretty great day, huh?" he said.

I nodded. It was.

"Yes." My knee screamed and I winced. "My knee is killing me. I'm going to look for a place to sit down. After I take one more picture." I snapped the picture. "I'm just glad to still be here."

Eric nodded. We held hands, everything tenuous and fragile. The year before, I had made a major scientific discovery that almost destroyed our family, and although I had succeeded in bringing Sebastian's unique neuroplastic adaptation to his vision impairment to the scientific community, I couldn't stop feeling scared.

***

"I can't help you, and I don't know anyone who can. Good luck with that!"

Dr. Liu's words echoed through my head, and I felt the wind knocked out of me. Dr. Liu's face was an unpleasant mask of barely concealed disgust. My face felt frozen. I was speechless as I slowly turned and looked at Sebastian. His face mirrored mine. Silently we walked together, following our disapproving escort through the long path back. It was a long and awkward walk, and Dr. Liu didn't say goodbye.

In the elevator on the way down, Sebastian said, "Welp, that didn't go well."

Our eyes met. I don't know what he saw, but I saw despair. I reached out and took his hand.

"It's okay," I said with more confidence than I felt. "We'll get this figured out."

"She told me I just need to do some visualization exercises," Sebastian said, disgustedly. "Like I haven't spent my entire fucking life trying to figure out how to picture things." His eyes and face were hard with fury. He punched his hand against the wall.

I had seen my son sad. I had seen my son frustrated and scared. This was the first time I had ever seen him furious, and I understood his rage. For his entire life, Sebastian had been telling us he needed help, and no one understood. I certainly hadn't understood, and neither had Eric. Once again, the person who should have helped him had failed him.

"Visualization exercises," Sebastian said bitterly and scoffed. "What an idiot."

I silently agreed, but I gave him the mom look anyway. He was sitting hunched and glowering out the car window.

"What can you visualize?" I asked him softly. I was afraid to ask, I realized. I was afraid to know. I held my breath, almost wishing he wouldn't answer.

Sebastian thought a moment. "Words," he said simply. "And letters." He looked sad as I snuck a glance at him beside me. He turned his eyes away from mine and thought a moment. "Numbers, too," he added. He paused again, considering, and without looking at me said, "And simple shapes."

The breath I had been holding escaped in a hard gasp. I sat, feeling paralyzed, with my hands on the steering wheel of the car. I couldn't look at him. I struggled to inhale.

"Anything else?" I finally choked out. "I mean, like, I can picture the Mona Lisa." I caught a quick glimpse as I said it; the long, dark hair, the lumpy cheeks, the heavy-lidded eyes. "It's a very fleeting image, but it's sharp, as long as I don't try to focus too much on the details."

Sebastian's face was fascinated, filled with wonder. He shook his head. "I can't do that."

"Can you take a circle and make it into a smiley face?"

"No," he said firmly. "I've tried a billion times. I can't."

"Maybe you could try rehearsing it?" I asked tentatively. "Like as an exercise? Maybe just, like, ten minutes a day? Maybe with repetition, that would help?"

Sebastian turned and pierced me with his eyes.

"I've been trying all my life, Mom," he said, in that way he does when he is absolutely, positively right. *Which is often,* I thought to myself. No one had spent more time drawing faces than Sebastian. If that didn't help him to recognize a face, I didn't know what would. I was struggling to process this new piece of information. I was having trouble even imagining what his vision must be like.

I burst out, "What is seeing like for you?"

His face softened as he considered. His eyes lost the bitter edge that made him look much older than his fifteen years.

"It's like being in an alien world where nothing ever looks familiar," he said simply. "Except for words, letters, numbers, and simple shapes."

I gripped the steering wheel hard, feeling the smooth plastic under my fingers. I tried to process. I looked through the windshield at the stores and gas stations passing by. I tried to imagine his visual world. I heard his words, but I couldn't understand. I felt terrified, too scared to imagine what he saw.

I intellectually understood the meaning of his words, but I couldn't imagine it. *I don't want to imagine it,* I thought to myself. *It is too terrifying to imagine, and so I won't.* My inner watcher shied away. I felt the hair on my arms, stiff. Ice water ran against gravity up my arms and back, across my scalp.

There is a stranger in my car, I thought. I saw him; his profile was in my peripheral vision. *I don't know my son. I only know the light that he reflects. My son is a chameleon, camouflaged so well that I have barely seen him.* His changeling skin was shedding off, in bits and pieces, and I was frightened for my child in a way I had never imagined possible.

My child was fifteen years old and I knew nothing important about him. I had only seen his surface; the shiny scales of artistic ability and academic accomplishment always glowed brilliantly. His sweet, gentle personality and especially his humor was a changing rainbow of color infusing everything. His anxiety must have been a tsunami, I realized, underneath the skin of perfection.

And then I had it: A tsunami. Like a science-fiction movie, some alternative universe where everything constantly changes, where there was no visual constant. Sebastian's visual world had no visual solidity, no nothing. I heard his voice: "Only words and letters, numbers, simple shapes."

I saw the sign for Main Street and in my mind's eye, it stood in sharp relief. M A I N S T floated past me, unattached to any object. It was its own reality.

I pulled over in the Meineke lot, shaking. In my imagination I could see this kaleidoscope of colors, changing swirls and blurs, never settling, never condensing. M E I N E K E. It floated suspended in the maelstrom. D U N K I N D O N U T S floated nearby. A tsunami of colors and unrecognizable shapes surrounded me. I saw through my child's eyes, and I was broken, undone.

My previous understanding of his lack of recognition of his environment was swept away in the tide of understanding. I got it. I saw it. I sat beside a mind so brilliant that even this total visual chaos had not prevented him from anything. Not only had he not been prevented, he had surmounted every challenge. I was speechless.

"Mom?" Sebastian asked. "Are you okay, Mom?"

"You are a miracle," I gasped.

He stared at me. "Are you okay, Mom?"

"I understand it!" I exhaled. "I see it. I understand how you've been seeing." I turned to him. "I know how scared you've been. I know how awful it has been for you."

Sebastian's anxiety had only ever made ripples in the thick perfection of his changeling outer skin, misunderstood, even though he plainly told us. I heard his voice that summer before sixth grade perfectly in my memory: "I'm afraid of getting lost, Mom."

"Why?" I asked, sitting in the therapist's office and wanting so badly to understand, to help. "Why are you so scared? I just don't understand."

"I don't know."

Of course he didn't know. He couldn't know because he'd never seen with a brain that saw. He couldn't know what he'd never experienced. He didn't know he was different. Perfect grades. Perfect friends. Perfect manners. Perfect child. All this perfection camouflaged perfectly this severely visually impaired child.

I went over in my head all the things of which I was certain. I knew my son had spent his entire life asking for help in the only way he knew how. Crying is communication. It tells you there's something wrong. He had been communicating his need for help for as long as he had been alive, and no one understood. I didn't understand, and certainly not his doctor or any of his teachers.

I can't blame them, I thought to myself. *I lived with this child for fifteen years and I couldn't tell he was severely visually impaired. There was no possible way Dr. Fredericks could pick up in a twenty-minute appointment what took me fifteen years of daily contact to discover.* I could not point a finger, except at myself. The guilt was overwhelming.

I tried, I know, but not enough, I realized. I vacillated between self-recrimination and knowing there was nothing that I could have done. From Dr. Liu's reaction, I knew Sebastian's agnosia was very rare. It said so when I Googled it, I reminded myself. It was a very small comfort. I couldn't stop going over what I could have done better and what I missed.

When Sebastian was little, I pointed out his separation anxiety to his doctor and his teachers, and they all told me he was fine.

"He settles quickly after drop-off," one told me, "He'll get used to it."

"It's the ones who have the temper tantrums that you need to be concerned about," another said, reassuring and confident. "Those are the ones you have to watch. He'll settle in, just you wait."

Not wanting to be "that mom," I shrugged off my niggling worries.

"Not to worry," they said. "Some kids just do this. He'll be fine."

Now I knew Sebastian was definitely not fine, and I was scared. At night I lay restlessly, and then got up and went downstairs. I paced the floor. Sebastian alone. Sebastian lost. Sebastian in danger. The next day I called Lukas at the Seeing Eye.

"Hi Lukas, it's Stephanie Duesing, Sebastian's mom, again."

Lukas greeted me kindly, his calm, baritone voice curious as I hesitated. He waited patiently for me to explain the reason for my call.

"I know this is a crazy idea," I hedged. I swallowed. "But, umm..." I sat down, and then stood again. "I, uh..." I pictured

Sebastian standing alone in Chicago, lost and terrified, cars swirling around him and strangers passing him on every side, blind to his vision impairment. "You know..." I took a breath and continued, "I was wondering... I know that the guide dog's owner has to completely trust the dog's judgment." I sat down again and rubbed my forehead. "But, ummm..." The next words came rushing out: "Could a dog ever be trained to be the navigator, if the person isn't able?"

I swallowed and then stood up and went to the window and looked out. Sebastian, alone out there, lost. "Like, maybe with a Garmin or something?"

Lukas, miraculously, didn't laugh. With deep compassion, kindness, and humor, he talked me down out of my crazy tree. He had a ready answer, and so afterwards I thought I probably wasn't the first to ask. It was a comfort.

***

"I will not allow another repeat of yesterday," I whispered to Sebastian as we sat waiting to see his new art therapist. It was the third of February, and Sebastian looked relieved. He'd had a multi-hour audiology assessment that morning, and now he was sitting in the waiting room with his paints and brushes. He was looking forward to meeting his new psychologist.

"I am coming in this time, right from the start. It's ridiculous how some adults have no faith in teenagers."

My nerves were still jangled from the appointment with Dr. Liu, and I fervently prayed today would go better. The auburn-haired receptionist with the multiple piercings called Sebastian's name, and Dr. Andrei S. Bucholz opened the door and flashed his dimples. His curly red hair was neat and nicely styled, and his soft green cardigan was casual yet professional-looking. He was kind and fatherly as we sat down. He took his shoes off and then invited us to do the same.

I explained everything we had discovered about Sebastian's face blindness, the environmental agnosia, and how we discovered it. I showed Dr. Bucholz the gap in Sebastian's scores on the WISC assessment and said I was certain the genius IQ had masked a serious visual-spatial deficit, leading to a false positive in his visual-spatial scores. Dr. Bucholz was quite surprised, but to his credit he recovered quickly. He was madly scribbling notes down when both his auburn eyebrows shot up and he abruptly stopped. He looked up at me, pen frozen in the air above his notepad.

"My colleague, Dr. Amanda Sturgis! She's had patients with agnosia before."

Sebastian and I looked at each other in surprise and relief.

"Is it okay if I bring her in to consult?"

"Yes!" Sebastian and I said in unison, and then smiled at each other.

"Great!" Dr. Bucholz opened a cabinet and produced the necessary releases, which I quickly signed. He sent a text while I filled out the forms, and just moments later there was a soft knock on the door.

"Come in!" Dr. Bucholz called.

Dr. Amanda Sturgis was about my age, and fit. Her athletic build was slender, and she moved gracefully across the small room to shake our hands. She seated herself in the only chair remaining by the door and looked at us expectantly, her long dark hair pulled back into a very messy ponytail. I was acutely aware we had only an hour-long appointment and were more than fifteen minutes into our allotted time. My words came out in a rush, trying to catch Dr. Sturgis up on what had happened.

Dr. Bucholz handed her the neuro psych evaluation and Dr. Sturgis paged through it quickly, looking shocked.

"The agnosia happened because of the concussion?" Dr. Sturgis asked, confused. She winked at me as she looked up.

I recoiled slightly, and then realized it was a tic.

"No!" I corrected her immediately. "I think he was born this way, and he's been compensating so well that it's been concealed." I pointed out the WISC scores and explained it all again. Dr. Sturgis listened, fascinated, and then without a word, she abruptly stood and walked out of the room.

"Was it something I said?" I looked at Dr. Bucholz in surprise.

"She's a unique individual," Dr. Bucholz said dryly. He noticed my expression and the professional mask slipped back on. He raised his eyebrows and looked down. "But she's very, very nice." He shuffled the papers on his desk, and then picked up the conversation where we left off.

Sebastian and I went through everything we could remember about how we discovered the agnosia and the subtle signs we missed. Dr. Bucholz took copious notes and said little.

"...and we don't even know if Sebastian will be able to drive," I finished. Sebastian looked down at the floor, and I looked from him to Dr. Bucholz. The hair on my arms stood up tall every time I thought of him on his own. "We've got to get him some help learning to navigate. He's going to college in just two years, and we know now he's been counting his steps and turns in our own home all this time. He can't live independently without some orientation and mobility training."

Dr. Bucholz nodded and added a few notes to his pad. He glanced at his watch and said regretfully, "Our time is up, unfortunately. We will have to continue this at our next session." He stood and handed me my coat. "This is fascinating," he smiled at Sebastian, "and we'll get it worked out." He turned back to me with a genuine smile. "Do you have your next appointment scheduled?"

I put on my winter jacket. "Yes, I have the next three on the calendar."

"That's perfect."

We shook hands all around and Sebastian and I headed out into the cold afternoon.

"That went better than I expected," Sebastian said, his face cautious.

"It couldn't have been worse than yesterday." I snuck a glance at him. "I just wish we had more information about this. I feel like we do all the talking, and no one says anything."

Sebastian nodded. The wind was freezing as we walked

through the parking lot towards the car. I pulled my zipper up higher and stuffed my hands into my pockets. A laugh bubbled up out of nowhere.

"At least they believed us."

Sebastian laughed too. "I felt like a criminal yesterday. Like an escapee from Alcatraz or something. I'm really glad we came today."

I unlocked the car and looked at him.

"Thank you, Mom, for doing this."

"Of course." I said. "That's my job." I smiled at him. "Thank you for being so appreciative, though. You are my heart, you know. I kind of like you and would like to keep you around for a while, and not have you get hit by a bus."

He grimaced, "Me, too." He started to get in the car.

"Wait!" a voice cried. "Wait!" I turned and saw Dr. Bucholz waving madly. "Wait!" He was running after us in his sock feet, dodging the slick icy patches. "Wait! Come back!"

Three-Hour Ride

"Come back!" Dr. Bucholz pulled his cardigan around himself and shouted, "Dr. Sturgis found her prosopagnosia face blindness test!"

Sebastian and I looked at each other, eyes huge.

"What?" We exclaimed simultaneously.

"Dr. Sturgis found her prosopagnosia test for the face blindness," Dr. Bucholz called again, hopping on his toes on the frozen asphalt. "Can you stay to be tested?"

An enormous rush of tension in my back and spine evaporated. Sebastian slammed the car door and ran around beside me. We grabbed hands and hope flooded Sebastian's face.

"Yes!" we cried as one.

Sebastian and I grinned foolishly at each other, and I one-arm hugged him as we walked back into the office. Even under his puffy winter jacket, he was so tall and slender. Dr. Bucholz danced on his tiptoes on the icy pavement and clutched his sweater against the bitter cold as we followed him back in. I gave silent thanks to God.

Dr. Sturgis was seated at Dr. Bucholz's desk when we returned. She had maneuvered her ponytail into a spectacular web of tangles on the top of her head and had a professionally bound spiral flipbook on the desk in front of her. She winked disconcertingly at Sebastian and indicated for him to sit across from her.

Sebastian shot me a look as he sat. I twitched my lip and then sat on the other chair right beside him. Dr. Bucholz seated himself in the chair by the door, taking notes.

The prosopagnosia face blindness test was very unusual-looking. Dr. Sturgis explained that Sebastian would need to look at one black-and-white photo of a person and then choose a match from six different photos below. The six photos in the line across the bottom of each page showed different facial expressions, lighting, and angles. The faces in the photos appeared almost contorted. They were striking in their harsh lighting and deep shadows.

I could see this was not an easy task. I could not see the differences among the faces from my seat right beside Sebastian. There were two parts to the test and in one of them, Sebastian was asked to pick out three photos of the same person from the six choices.

Sebastian sat, looking very carefully at each set of photos. My perfectionist child was concentrating hard in a way I had never, ever seen him do. I had seen him concentrated and focused on his art more times than I could count, but this was different. He was struggling to solve a puzzle, which astounded me. He examined the first page for a long time and then carefully, he made his first choice. Dr. Bucholz recorded the response in his notes.

One by one, page by page, Sebastian slowly and carefully went through both sections of the test. I watched with a mixture of concern and incredulity. This was the first time in my life I had ever seen him challenged by anything, ever. It was shocking to watch him struggle through the test. It took some time, and when it was over, I could see he was exhausted from the effort. He looked at me.

"That was hard." Sebastian sagged back into his chair, his face wan and pale. The concussion headache raged across his features. I squeezed his hand.

"You did great. Are you okay?"

"Ummhmm." He rubbed his head and heaved a sigh. "I'm fine, just tired."

Dr. Bucholz tallied up Sebastian's score and shared it with Dr. Sturgis. Dr. Sturgis's eyes widened. She winked, glanced at Sebastian, and then looked back down at the scores, shaking her head. She looked up at me, eyes wide.

"He scored significantly below impaired." Dr. Sturgis looked again at Sebastian, shock on her face, and then at me.

All my attention was on my son. His face was working: panic, surprise, frustration. I saw him rocketing from one emotion to another: grief, frustration, relief, fear, hope, confusion. I grabbed his hand as he turned to me, feeling his cool fingers in my own warm hand.

Sebastian's face went completely blank. He slumped back in his chair. I didn't know what he was feeling. I wanted to comfort him, to tell him everything would be okay, but I couldn't find the words. All the panic of the last few days had been overwhelming. The idea of my child, lost in the world, blind and helpless, had haunted my every waking moment. I could only imagine what Sebastian was feeling, and I knew it wasn't good.

I felt my heart surge with gratitude as I looked at the two doctors marveling over the test results. I could feel the fear for Sebastian's future, not leaving, but pulling back, receding. The wild panic of the past ten days subsided to a gnawing anxiety.

I was simultaneously exhausted and uplifted. Physically, I was tired. I had barely slept since the day of the photos, I realized suddenly. My nose was still drippy from crying earlier and I reached for the box of tissues on the desk. I looked with gratitude around the room. I could tell we were lucky to have found these two doctors, because everyone looked as shocked as I felt.

Dr. Bucholz was reading through the neuro psych report, shaking his head in amazement. Dr. Sturgis was going over the prosopagnosia face-blindness scores again intently. She glanced at her watch.

"It's almost five," she said, her eyes wide with surprise. She winked at me again, and I pretended not to notice.

"We have been here for three hours!" I stretched, legs stiff from sitting, and yawned. "No wonder I'm so tired."

Sebastian sat silently, staring down at nothing. He was so far away, he felt unreachable. I felt words rising in my throat as I reached towards him when Dr. Bucholz interrupted, concerned.

"Did you get in with the psychiatrist, Dr. Sheltze?"

"Yes," I said. "We had our intake, but Sebastian doesn't see him until the twenty-second."

Dr. Bucholz nodded.

"It was the first available," I explained, shrugging helplessly. Sebastian's appointment was almost three weeks away, and it felt like decades. I looked at Sebastian, disengaged. Silent.

"Do you think it's safe to leave him unmedicated until the twenty-second?" Dr. Bucholz asked.

"No." The answer came out without hesitation, surprising me.

Finally, Sebastian looked at me. Devastation. *He knows now he's really different from his friends,* I thought. *He knows he probably will never drive. He knows he may not go to college or live on his own.* I wanted to swoop him in my arms and hold him in my lap like when he was small, and cradle him and keep him safe. Instead I looked on helplessly. A flutter of panic rose and then settled again as Dr. Sturgis explained that there was an anti-anxiety medication called Effexor.

"It's a non-serotonin medication," she said. "Many of our patients use it."

"It's very safe," Dr. Bucholz assured me, seeing my hesitation. "Just take him to your primary care physician to get him started."

"Dr. Fredericks doesn't feel comfortable prescribing psychotropic meds to children," I reminded him. "Remember what happened with Dr. Marshall and the Lexapro? The ER doctor had to call poison control. Sebastian may have a genetic liver enzyme deficiency or difference in processing medications. We are having the genetic testing done on the twenty-second with Dr. Sheltze."

Dr. Bucholz lifted one reddish eyebrow and nodded slightly. "Well, Effexor is a non-serotonin medication, so you won't have to worry about him having serotonin syndrome again."

"It was very scary. He stopped breathing from the spasms."

"Don't worry. I will call Dr. Fredericks myself and explain what's going on." Dr. Bucholz smiled. "Just give me one day."

I heaved a sigh. "Thank you!" It was Friday, I realized. "Dr. Fredericks has Saturday hours. Do you mean you will call her tomorrow?" I looked at Sebastian, silent and slumped further in his chair. I was feeling more concerned for him by the second.

"Yes." Dr. Bucholz's smile was fatherly and warm. My whole

body relaxed.

"Thank you." I looked at Dr. Sturgis and smiled at her, too. "Thank you both so, so much. You are such a blessing. We can't tell you what a relief it is that we found you both."

"You are very welcome." Dr. Bucholz's freckled face dimpled charmingly.

He quickly found the release forms for me to sign so that he could speak with Dr. Fredericks about the Effexor. My obnoxiously large and loopy signature felt exhausting and I was ready to go home. We stood, exchanging smiles and handshakes. Sebastian stirred. He rubbed his face and rejoined the world.

"Call the office tomorrow and schedule the rest of the agnosia testing," Dr. Sturgis said, rising lightly from her chair and slipping quietly out the door.

"I will," I replied to her back, surprised and grateful there was more help coming. "Thank you both so much, again," I said rather loudly to both doctors, as one was already out the door. The door clicked shut behind Dr. Sturgis. "My friend was right," I said to Dr. Bucholz. "You really are amazing."

Over dinner Sebastian and I filled Eric in on everything that had happened, and then on Saturday morning I called Dr. Sturgis's office as instructed and scheduled the rest of the agnosia testing for the next Friday at 9 a.m. I thought about how we had joked about giving Sebastian my car to drive last fall. Everything was different now. The courage of this child stunned me, and also saddened me beyond any words. That he had had to figure out his own way of navigating all by himself as a toddler was unbearable.

Eric told me he was thinking about joining another pool league and playing two nights a week. He would have pool on Sunday and Wednesday evenings now, and he usually practiced with friends on Saturday afternoons. I was happy he was enjoying it so much, but I couldn't help feeling like he was distancing himself during a difficult time.

I was envious of Eric's ability to just act like everything was normal and simultaneously aware that having both of us stewing at home wasn't going to help things. Plus, Eric had worked so hard over the years. He had added an MBA to his other master's degree when Sebastian was two and he did so much for us both at work and at home. I encouraged Eric to join.

***

On Monday morning, I took a moment before Sebastian got up to check out the Effexor Dr. Sturgis had recommended for Sebastian's anxiety. Since the two of us each have drug allergies, plus our experience with the Lexapro, I was always cautious about all medications. I consulted Dr. Google and was surprised and concerned to discover that Effexor is not a non-serotonin medication as Dr. Sturgis had said. I thought perhaps I had recalled the wrong name, so I checked the handwritten note that Dr. Sturgis gave me. It was Effexor she had recommended.

It's just a mix-up, I thought, as I refilled my coffee. *Dr. Sturgis probably meant to suggest a medication with a similar name.* I was about to send her an email message for clarification when Sebastian came down for breakfast. He looked unwell. His normally fair skin was white and dark circles smudged bluish underneath his eyes.

"I woke up flat on my face on the carpet last night." He nodded towards the middle of the family room floor. "I was like this." He spread his arms out wide to the side, Christ-like. He had the same sad eyes. My scalp prickled.

"Really?" I asked. This was new information. "Your dad was a sleepwalker, and I caught you sleepwalking once when you were two or three, just after we bought this house. Has this happened before?"

"Yeah." He thought. "A couple of times."

My heart rate rose. I looked at his face carefully. He was more pale than usual, with dark shadows under his eyes.

"How many times?" I asked. "Where were you going?"

I pictured him wandering out the patio doors, across Moby Deck, and tumbling down the stairs. Or worse, not tumbling, and walking through the midnight quiet of the neighborhood. The hairs on my arm prickled to match my scalp. Bellini's "Ah! Non credea mirarti" began involuntarily in my internal soundtrack.

"Nowhere, really," he replied quickly, picking up on my anxiety, sensitive to my feelings, as he always is. *How does he do that,* I wondered for the millionth time, *if he can't recognize my face? How does he recognize the feelings? There is no question that he does, and always has.*

"A couple times I woke up with my nose to the refrigerator." He laughed, but not with amusement.

I laughed, too, sort off. I felt goosebumps prick up my arms again. How terrifying to wake up and have no idea where you are, and to not be able to see. I swallowed and stilled my face.

"That must have been really weird."

Sebastian was watching my face attentively. He nodded.

"It was." He paused. "I didn't know where I was at first, until I felt the handle."

I wanted to gather him into my arms like a toddler and hold him. Instead I said, "That must have been terrifying. Were you scared?"

I imagined myself waking up somewhere and having no idea where I was, and not able to see either. Panic swirled in my veins and I looked sharply at Sebastian's face. I exhaled, trying to calm myself. He watched me carefully, not answering.

I asked again. "Were you okay?"

He looked down. "Yeah, I was fine." He fiddled with the blanket. "I figured out where I was really quick."

I need to tell Dr. Bucholz, I thought. The agnosias, the memory problems, the depression, the drug reactions, and now sleepwalking. It sounded like Lewy body dementia. I breathed deeply. *All of Sebastian's brain scans for the concussion came back normal,* I told myself. *If there was a tumor, they would have seen it.* I stilled my face.

"Let's get a Starbucks on the way to school," I suggested.

***

I sent a polite email message through the proper channels to Dr. Bucholz with my concerns about Sebastian's drug reactions, asked whether the Effexor was the correct medication, and shared the new information about the sleepwalking. I asked for a phone call to discuss Sebastian's case before his appointment with Dr. Fredericks for anti-anxiety medications the next day. Then I checked my calendar for the day.

I was completely taken by surprise to see I had a physical that day. I had forgotten all about it with everything going on. Best of all, the appointment was with Dr. Fredericks. I was relieved to talk to this amazing doctor whom I had trusted for more than twenty years. I decided I would ask if I could use my appointment time to fill her in what had been going on with Sebastian.

Dr. Fredericks's white-streaked waves of brown hair lay neatly around her shoulders, and her gold frames glinted as she greeted me. Her large green eyes were filled with their usual kindness and curiosity as she sat. I was so filled with relief that I just launched into our story: Sebastian not recognizing faces, navigating like a blind person, Dr. Bucholz and Dr. Sturgis and the severely impaired score on the face-blindness test. The story just tumbled out of me like a tidal wave. When I looked up, Dr. Fredericks was staring at me like I was a lunatic.

"Wait," she said. "Who are these people?"

Box of Kittens

Heat crept up my already flushed face. I felt a horrible sense of panic rising, and tears started. The stress of the last few days took over and I couldn't hold back the grief any longer.

"Dr. Andrei Bucholz?" I stared at Dr. Fredericks, willing her to recognize the name. "He said he would call you."

Dr. Fredericks watched me with concern, thought a moment, then frowned and shook her head. "No," she said carefully. "I don't know anything about this."

I couldn't help it. I started to cry in earnest. Dr. Fredericks quickly handed me tissues and asked me who was supposed to call. I explained everything, and Dr. Fredericks kindly took me back to her private office and called Dr. Bucholz's office herself, in my presence. Neither Dr. Bucholz nor Dr. Sturgis was available, so Dr. Fredericks asked for a call back. She left her name and number, then hung up.

"You are coming back tomorrow with Sebastian?"

I nodded.

"Good. We'll talk some more tomorrow."

She was polite but distant, and I got up to go. I felt very disturbed by the lack of follow-through from Dr. Bucholz, and I was so embarrassed and uncomfortable that I didn't even think to stay for my physical. The rest of the day went by in jumble of fear. I got no phone call or return email messages from either Dr. Bucholz or Dr. Sturgis.

I took Sebastian in to see Dr. Fredericks as scheduled the next day, which was Tuesday, February 3rd. My internal alarms were blaring. I hadn't heard from either Dr. Bucholz or Dr. Sturgis regarding the Effexor, and for the very first time in over twenty years, I was uncomfortable with Dr. Fredericks.

She came into the exam room looking deeply skeptical and uncomfortable. Her eyes looked sad and slightly hostile behind the gold-framed glasses. She watched my reactions with suspicion, and then said she hadn't gotten a return phone call from either doctor. Her eyes regarded me with deep pity and concern.

The more I tried to explain to her, the more she looked skeptical, and obviously concerned for my mental health. Dr. Fredericks had known Sebastian since he was two, and he didn't look at all blind in any of the interactions she had had with him for thirteen years. She didn't say it, but it was obvious she thought I was nuts.

I forged on anyway, laying out everything we discovered as calmly as I could. I explained my concerns, and medicating Sebastian for his anxiety. She refused to prescribe any anti-anxiety medication for Sebastian, as I knew she would, and as I had clearly explained twice to Dr. Bucholz.

"Sebastian can wait until he sees the psychiatrist on February 22," she said. She checked her calendar. "It's only seventeen days away."

I strongly but politely disagreed with her. Sebastian was really struggling. He was withdrawing more and more every second. I asked for a referral to a specialist for neurological visual impairment and she refused.

"I don't think it's necessary," Dr. Fredericks said.

The whole appointment was extremely awkward and uncomfortable. I decide to self-refer to a major neurology clinic in southern California. One of my Musikgarten moms had taken her father there for a rare brain tumor the previous year. I had the doctor's card this mom had given me in my purse.

It was after four o'clock on Wednesday, February 8, and I was driving home from the medical records office when my phone rang. I pulled over to a side street and answered it. It was Dr. Bucholz. He was cool and distant.

"What happened?" I demanded. "You said you would call Dr. Fredericks. Why didn't you call like you said you were going to?"

"I'm sorry I didn't get back to you," he said impersonally. "I put Sebastian's case up for a meeting with our director."

I inhaled sharply. "I didn't give you permission to discuss his case with anyone other than Dr. Fredericks. What is going on here?"

"Well," Dr. Bucholz said coyly, "we didn't use any names, so it's permissible."

I was angry but controlled. "You realize Dr. Fredericks thinks I'm a lunatic now. She had no idea what I was talking about. Do you have any idea how that feels? She's known Sebastian since he was two years old. I looked completely crazy going in there saying Sebastian is blind and that you were going to call her. She's been my doctor for more than twenty years! I feel like you destroyed my relationship with my own doctor."

"I'm sorry you feel that way," he replied in his detached, clinical tone. "When Dr. Fredericks called, the message went to Dr. Sturgis, and you didn't sign a release for her to speak with Dr. Fredericks."

Yeah, this is my fault, I thought sarcastically. "I signed the release form for *you* to speak with her, and *you* said you were going to call her *on Saturday*," I replied, biting my words off crisply. "Not Tuesday." *Or today*, I thought, but I kept myself from saying it out loud.

"Well, the meeting with the director wasn't until this afternoon," Dr. Bucholz said smoothly. Then with very fake concern, like he was speaking to an unreasonable child, he said, "That's why I'm calling now."

I sat back in my seat. "I am taking Sebastian to Southern California to the neurology center there."

He paused, surprised. "Please wait. You don't need to take him now."

"Yes, I do. Sebastian needs help now."

"Please don't do this. You can wait and take him in January of next year."

"January? Are you kidding me? That's a year from now. No," I said firmly. "He is having major neurological issues now. He's already got a very late discovery of his disability. Our time is short to access services. He's already fifteen. He needs help now."

"He can wait. It's just a year."

What is he freaked out about? I wondered. "No. I already faxed the records."

That stopped him short. His tone changed abruptly. "I'd like you to come in without Sebastian on Thursday to discuss his case," he said.

"Okay," I agreed. "That's fine."

We set up an appointment time and ended the call. A few minutes later Dr. Fredericks called. She very patiently and with exaggerated reasonableness explained that she was "the coordinator of Sebastian's care." She said that "agnosia is something that many people have, and it's just something that people learn to cope with." She said, "Sebastian doesn't need a diagnosis for his IEP."

I strongly but politely disagreed.

On Thursday, February 9, I went in to see Dr. Bucholz. Sebastian wanted to come, but I told him Dr. Bucholz specifically asked to see me alone to discuss his case. It was weird and we both knew it. Sebastian was upset by this news and so was I.

When I arrived, Dr. Bucholz was cool and distant. He asked me if it was okay to include Dr. Fredericks in the meeting.

"It's a little late now," I said, pointedly. "You said you were going to call her on Saturday."

Dr. Bucholz's expression didn't change and he didn't reply.

"Yes, you may include Dr. Fredericks, as she is the coordinator of Sebastian's care."

Dr. Bucholz called Dr. Fredericks on her cell and put her on speakerphone. After the greetings, he said, "Because Sebastian had some visual memory testing done in December for the concussion, for legal and ethical reasons he shouldn't have had the agnosia testing so soon afterwards."

"Why?" I asked, incredulous. "What is the big deal?"

"Because it's a visual memory test," he explained. "Once you see it, you can never take it again."

I sat back and folded my arms, my voice clipped. "Why was the face-blindness test given if it's not allowed?"

Dr. Bucholz shifted his eyes uncomfortably and looked past me at the wall behind me, not meeting my eyes. "We were just trying to help."

I felt my incredulity rising as I stared at his smooth mask of a face. He looked down at his papers and shuffled a page.

He's acting like he botched a surgery, I thought. *Like he amputated the wrong leg. Are they really so afraid the doctors at the neurology center in Southern California will see he made a glorified clerical error? Does he think we're going to sue them?* I stared at him, incredulous.

"What is the big deal?" I asked, confused and alarmed. As kindly as I could, I said, "We are grateful for the testing. We aren't complaining."

"It's a legal issue," Dr. Bucholz replied, his face too still.

"We aren't suing you," I told him, even more incredulously. "We are glad we found you. We don't care that you made a minor error!" *Why would he think this of us? Did we not express our gratitude effusively?* I pleaded with him, "Sebastian has to have a diagnosis for the school."

Dr. Fredericks's alto voice interjected calmly from Dr. Bucholz's cell phone. "It's okay. I can attend Sebastian's IEP meeting and we can just give him a general label."

"No!" I said. Everything Patty Kelly told me came right out. "A general label will not get him the vision services he needs. Services like orientation and mobility disappear dangerously for people over age twenty-two who have visual disabilities, and at age fifteen, Sebastian has had a very late diagnosis already." I continued, not relenting. "He should have had O&M training years ago," I argued. "He does not have the skills to live independently, to go to college or to safely drive."

Very calmly and patiently, like I was more than a little slow and extremely unreasonable, Dr. Fredericks's disembodied alto voice came out of the cell phone. She said, "Agnosia is extremely common and just something that people learn to deal with without help."

I could not believe what I was hearing. I sat there, stunned.

"That's ridiculous," I said, my voice tight. "Sebastian needs O&M. We aren't asking for narcotics; we are asking for some basic services for him. Sebastian is smart. He probably only needs a few weeks of lessons in navigation. I don't understand why this is so difficult."

"Thank you, Dr. Fredericks." Dr. Bucholz turned his cold eyes on mine. "I am going to hang up now." He ended the call and looked dismissively at me. "I am going to discontinue care for Sebastian," Dr. Bucholz stated flatly, "before the therapist bond is created."

He stood. I was dismissed. My heart stopped. I sat there, my head shaking, not understanding. Dr. Bucholz stood at the open door silently. I stood and walked towards him, completely lost.

"It's too late," I told him truthfully. "He's already bonded."

The old sense of falling off the planet from so long ago engulfed me. My hair prickled up my arms, my neck, and across my head. Dr. Bucholz stood firmly holding the door, eyes disapproving, and lips compressed. Desperately, I tried again.

"Are you serious? Sebastian begged me to come today," I pleaded. "Please don't do this! Sebastian really likes you. I don't know what he'll do. We need your help. We know he has lasting trauma from going undiagnosed for so many years. I think he may have PTSD from having to teach himself to count his steps and turns." I took a breath. "We need you."

Dr. Bucholz's face was stiff and cold, his eyes hard. The unreality of the situation made everything seem like a funhouse mirror. I was watching everything that unfolded like it was a movie, but oddly distorted in time and slowed-down. I was standing in the doorway, begging a doctor for help. I stared at him, pleading with my eyes.

"No," he said flatly. "I can't. I'm not qualified." He stiffly ushered me out the door.

"I'm worried he might hurt himself. What am I going to do?"

Dr. Bucholz's face was stony. "I don't know. Goodbye."

He closed the door in my face. I cried the entire ride home. I had no idea what to tell Sebastian. My thoughts were just chaotic. I knew he was going to be devastated, rejected. He'd spent his entire life asking for help, and the first person to offer it had just dumped us like a box of kittens on a country road.

I needed to find another therapist, and quickly. At the red light at Main and First, I realized Dr. Bucholz didn't even give us a referral to another therapist. I sat in the car in the driveway for half an hour when I got home. I couldn't go in. I couldn't face Sebastian.

Telling Sebastian that Dr. Bucholz dropped us from his care was the saddest thing I have ever had to do, and I have put down two beloved dogs.

The following day Eric and I wrote a formal letter requesting all of Sebastian's records from Drs. Bucholz and Sturgis, including but not limited to notes, records, evaluations, and all test results. Eric faxed it to Dr. Bucholz's office at work the next day. I wondered if we would ever see the prosopagnosia face-blindness test results. I suspected we would not.

"Do you think we should see a lawyer?" I asked Eric, sitting uncomfortably and fidgeting. "I just think something is really wrong."

"No," he shook his head. "Those records are our property. They have to send them to us."

Eric was so stolid and had such faith in people's general goodness, which I think comes from being raised in such a nice family. I didn't feel reassured, though, and I sat down at the computer and began to document everything that was going on. I typed a long time, and I documented everything I could remember from our first appointment with Dr. Liu for the concussion.

Just days later, on Valentine's Day, February 14, 2017, we enrolled Sebastian in a day program for anxiety. Because of his drug reaction to Lexapro he couldn't be safely medicated until we saw his new psychiatrist on the twenty-second. Sebastian needed to have genetic testing done for a possible liver enzyme difference in processing medications, and he couldn't be medicated until after that time. Although he had never once verbally threatened anything, I was afraid for his life.

Every day I anxiously awaited news from the neurology clinic in Southern California. I hoped desperately that someone there had heard of this condition. I sent a detailed description of exactly how we discovered Sebastian's agnosias, and the way he'd been verbally compensating. I didn't understand exactly how Sebastian had been functioning as well as he was, but I knew it was with words. I knew Sebastian was recognizing verbal characteristics he had assigned things. And just like that, as I untangled memory after memory, I knew.

In my mind's eye, I saw him as a toddler, sitting at the kitchen table with Moby Deck behind him. Sebastian was two and a half and it was our first summer in this house. Sebastian was coloring Teletubbies. He had all the dolls around him, even NuuNuu, my personal favorite. He was coloring the TV screen in Tinky's tummy with a gray marker.

"What are you coloring?" I asked him.

"Tinky's TV screen," he said happily. "Tinky has a triangle," he informed me solemnly.

"Yes, he does," I said, echoing his tone.

"He's purple and has a triangle," Sebastian continued, coloring carefully in the lines as he spoke. "And Dipsy is green. He has a straight up!" He threw both arms straight up in the air joyously, so filled with toddler charm that I couldn't help grinning at his enthusiasm.

"Yes, he does," I agreed, amused. "He does have a straight up."

"Laa Laa is yellow, and she has a curlicue." He whirled his hand in a curlicue motion in the air with his marker. "And Po is red," he finished. "Po is red with a circle."

Purple + triangle = Tinky-Winky, I thought. There were hundreds of Teletubby pages Sebastian went through, and when he got bored coloring the pages, he drew his own. The memories came roaring back.

"Thumb!"

I heard the excitement in his little voice. I looked at Sebastian's coloring page. He was coloring Tinky's thumb and pointing at it, his eyes meeting mine, asking for my agreement.

Purple + triangle + head + ears + eyes + nose + mouth +

arms + hands + thumbs + legs + feet + TV screen = Tinky-Winky.

I saw the pattern.

"Yes, that is his thumb," I said. I was oblivious at the time to how miraculous it was that my child knew he was coloring a Teletubby thumb.

***

As I watched Sebastian going about his daily routine, now as a teenager, I noticed everything. I watched him getting silverware from the drawer, finding his backpack, and putting his laundry away. He stored his art supplies neatly in his art room.

There was so much I didn't understand about Sebastian's vision. I didn't know how it was possible he could ride a bike, or even run or walk without bumping into things. He had always, every quarter, gotten an A in gym. His gym teacher marked him as "very athletic" during the grade promotion process.

I could barely plan my choir lessons, and my Musikgarten classes went by in a fog of faces. His blindness was just all impossible. Sebastian painted and drew with great skill for a high schooler.

I believed Sebastian when he said he could recognize only words, letters, numbers, and simple shapes. I saw with my own eyes his inability to recognize his own face. I saw his face light up with understanding when he touched his scarf on the table that night in the kitchen. I knew without a doubt he had face blindness and environmental blindness. I believed Sebastian also had object agnosia, but when I asked him how he recognized objects, he couldn't explain how he did it.

If Sebastian had object agnosia, that meant he was recognizing millions of ordinary objects by the way we describe them, not by how they look. His semantic memory would have to be immense, I decided. I couldn't wrap my mind around it, and so I observed, and we talked.

"Everything has characteristics," he told me again, matter-of-factly, as he bent over his drawing.

Waiting to hear from the neurology clinic felt like agony. I wondered a million times a day if we had any chance at all of getting in with a self-referral. Probably not, I decided. I couldn't leave things to chance, so when Sebastian slumped upstairs to take a nap, carting the laundry with him without me asking, I made an appointment with a local neurologist and a neuro ophthalmologist. It was almost a four-month wait for the neuro ophthalmologist, but I heard he was worth it.

That night I lay restlessly in bed and wondered what the next step was. I didn't know what to do. It was possible I was wrong about him being born with this vision thing. The thing that kept me up at night was his bird painting. I remembered it like it was yesterday; Sebastian in his booster chair and Penny eating Cheerios. Nickie tackling Penny and chewing gently on her little ears; Sebastian in my arms; the smell of banana in his hair, and him standing at his easel, painting. Sebastian turning to me and signing "bird." He recognized a bird shape before he could say the word "bird."

Maybe he wasn't born with this, I thought. Maybe it was something he was developing, perhaps accelerated by the concussion. I couldn't shake the niggling fear. The memory issues, sleepwalking, the depression, the visual perceptual difficulties, and the bizarre drug reaction, it was all so strange. I thought maybe he had some horrible, early-onset Lewy body dementia.

He had a CT scan for the concussion in October. It was unremarkable. *Was it possible he had something blooming we didn't know about?* I lay in bed and wondered. Maybe something was reaching soft, sticky fingers into his razor-sharp mind.

I couldn't sleep. I adjusted Big Squishy and rolled over for the third time in five minutes. Eric sighed, annoyed. He had early meetings with his India team almost every single day.

"I talked to Seb today," I said. "He said, 'Everything has characteristics,' and do you know what? Mine are tall/blonde/glasses." I didn't know why this small fact mattered to me so much, but I felt like I finally knew myself through my son's eyes.

"Hmmm." Eric pulled the covers higher.

"He's using words to recognize people," I continued. "Matt's characteristics are his freckles and his super thick brown hair. It stands straight up, like a brush." Eric's eyes opened. "I Googled it, and it's typical for people with face blindness to use other characteristics than facial features to recognize people. Like, even their gait!" I said, excitedly. "You know that one friend? That stands like a boxer?"

Eric nodded, "Yeah. What's his name? Jake?"

"Yeah!" I agreed. "That one. That's how Sebastian recognizes him, by the way he stands. And his bright red hair." I pulled the covers up a little higher and waited. Eric's face was thoughtful for a moment. I waited, expectantly. "Isn't that interesting?" I asked him, marveling at this new piece of information. I felt like a detective or a bloodhound, chasing down new clues. Sherlock Holmes. "Well?"

"Well," Eric said as he leaned up on his elbow to look down at me. "What I can't figure out is why he's lying about it."

Refrigerator Mother

I jerked myself upright with a hard shove and pushed the covers back. I sat up, staring at Eric's face in the dimly lit room. The moonlight from the skylight in the bathroom backlit him, making his expression impossible to decipher. I felt the cool air on my legs as I swung them out of bed and stood, turning to face him. I was bristling.

"Are you kidding me? Sebastian is not lying." I realized how loud that was, and I didn't know if Sebastian was asleep. *Probably not,* I thought. I lowered my voice and hissed, "What are you saying?"

Eric shrugged. "I just don't see how he could have this," he said flatly. "It just doesn't make any sense."

"Your son is not a liar," I said, spitting every word. I couldn't believe what I was hearing. I drew myself up to my full height and pointed at him. "Name one time he has ever told a lie."

That caught Eric off guard, and he blinked, his eyes gray in the moonlight. He knew it was the truth. Sebastian had never been in trouble. He had never been spanked; he had never once been grounded. He had never had a detention or been in trouble at a friend's house.

When we'd mentioned this fact to his therapist in middle school, she made one comment, "Hmmm... Abnormally compliant," and put it in her notes. When I asked why this should be, she simply frowned slightly and shrugged.

"You're right," Eric admitted. "He's not a liar. I've never caught him in a lie." He paused, considering. "You know, I've never even suspected he was hiding something."

"Well, he's been hiding quite a lot from us," I said, mollified. "Unwittingly. What must it be like to discover you are completely different than everyone you know, than everyone you've ever met?"

Eric rolled onto his back and looked up at the ceiling. I sighed.

"Jake got his driver's license today."

Eric said nothing. I saw Jake's smiling face, holding up his driver's license, his red hair brilliant and his smile even brighter. Damn Facebook.

Eric was so private, he didn't use Facebook at all. *Maybe he had the right idea,* I thought to myself, *but I would miss all the connections to my friends.*

"Thank God we discovered it before Sebastian started driver's ed."

"Mmmhmm." Eric rolled back over, pulling the covers up again.

It's weird how two people can see something so differently, I thought. In my imagination I saw Eric sitting in his favorite spot, watching TV with his noise-canceling headphones on. *He didn't see what I saw,* I comforted myself. *He didn't hear what I heard. I know he doesn't know what I know, but he believes me now, and Sebastian too.*

I climbed back in bed, flipped the Lunk over to the cool side, and mushed Big Squishy in a ball against my chest. Eric reached out and hugged me to him.

"I love you."

"I love you, too."

It will be okay, I thought. *We are on the same page now and we will get through this.*

***

A few days later we had an appointment at the Chicago Lighthouse to meet with the technology team for the blind and visually impaired. "Please come with us." I begged Eric at 5:45 that morning.

I had tried to interest Eric in attending the meeting a couple of times, but so much was happening at work, he told me. I knew he was stressed about one particular project especially that he was trying to keep from going off the rails. His group had a lot of deliverables coming up. He buttoned his cuffs and then put on his watch.

"It's a meeting with the technology team," I re-explained.

Eric shook his head slightly. "I really would like you to be there. There may be things that can help Sebastian navigate, and I'm not the technology expert in the family, you are."

"I have nine meetings today," he said, his lips tight. "I'll be home around six thirty."

I felt like crying as he went stomping down the stairs. But I didn't. I didn't cry. Instead I made butternut squash lasagna with a goat cheese béchamel.

Thank you, Fine Cooking, I thought, as I peeked in the deli drawer. *I did have goat cheese back there. It was almost like I planned it.* I celebrated the small things as I set the timer on the squash for fifty minutes.

When we arrived at the Lighthouse, the technology team met us right away. They were three vital men, energetic and filled with enthusiasm for their jobs. They clearly loved their work, and everyone was so kind and welcoming. The three of them bantered cheerfully back and forth with Sebastian.

I wanted to relax, and although everyone was very friendly and helpful, I kept waiting for them to demand a note from a doctor. I felt like an imposter, like they might kick us out at any moment. I kept waiting for some snide remark.

"And what is his diagnosis?" someone would say, with a knowing look around the table.

Instead, everyone was helpful and extremely kind and courteous. The three men were clearly interested and engaged in helping us. We chatted and they asked us what we needed.

I had no idea what was possible, so I said, "Everything."

They laughed and they demoed a new product for us. There were glasses that recognized faces from OrCam. They had a built-in camera and a speaker that talked to the person wearing them. It used facial-recognition software, the lead person explained.

One of the younger men put the glasses on to demonstrate for Sebastian.

"You must program in each person," the young man explained. The software couldn't recognize strangers, and sunglasses or hats could interfere with its ability to recognize even familiar faces. It was not a perfect solution, but the possibilities were exciting. I felt a surge of hopefulness.

"This could be really helpful for you." I said to Sebastian. He was paying close attention, but clearly not feeling this product was right for him. I was obviously more excited about it than he was.

We moved on to discuss iPhones and using Google Maps to navigate. There is a watch, they told me, that vibrates to tell the user when to turn right or left. I couldn't help it. The tears came.

"It's the shock," one gentleman said, with a kind glance around the table.

We were not alone. They had seen other people like us. I was a weepy mess as I looked at the kindly faces, all looking on so patiently and so understandingly. They had seen this all before, they knew the drill and they were used to moms like me. I was obviously not the first to cry. I glanced around as I tried to pull myself together. I avoided looking at their faces, because to see the compassion and understanding there would cause my wheels to fall off completely, I knew.

"Thank you," I said to no one in particular, and I quickly wiped my stupid eyes. *I am not bad for crying,* I told myself. *Anyone who was in this situation would.* "You must have read my message." They all nodded, and then they brought out more tech toys. It turns out there are all kinds of gadgets for people with visual impairments.

When it was time to go I had so much to think about and new hope that Sebastian could learn to find his way, even if he could never drive.

"Let us know when you are ready," one of them said. "We can take you all around the city and show you how to use Google Maps to get around." The three men looked ready to take us out right then and there. I felt a huge surge of relief and optimism as we all shook hands. We exchanged goodbyes and headed home.

At home, feeling better, Sebastian helped me finish the lasagna. He crumbled goat cheese while I filled a large pot of water and then brought it to a boil.

"What did you think about the glasses?" I asked Sebastian, trying to sound casual.

"I don't know," Sebastian said, nonplussed. "I don't think I really need them."

"Don't you think it might make things easier? I mean, at school?" I asked. "You could program all your friends in and then when you pass them in the hallway, you wouldn't miss them."

I pictured him passing swarms of other students in the halls. How many millions of times had he walked right past someone and not responded to a grin? I wondered how many times people had thought he was unfriendly or stuck up. His tight-knit group of friends was so faithful and sweet. I knew he wasn't perceived that way by those who knew and loved him. I felt a sudden surge of anger and sadness for him.

"I don't know," he said, shrugging. "The water's boiling. Do you want me to put in the lasagna?"

"Sure."

He grabbed the box of lasagna noodles and opened it, dumping the contents in the water. Then he put the empty carton in the recycle bin under the sink. I handed him a pasta stirrer from the drawer in front of me. He stirred the pasta and considered, his face inscrutable.

"Don't you think it would be easier if you had those glasses? Kids might think you are stuck up if you don't recognize them in the hall. I know they are a little bulkier than ordinary frames, and the camera is pretty obvious. Do you think they look too dorky?"

"Maybe. Did you salt the water?"

"No."

Sebastian opened the spice cabinet and grabbed the Morton's Salt box. He dumped a tablespoonful into his palm and tossed it into the steaming pot.

"I just think it would be easier for you if you knew who the people were around you."

"I usually do, Mom. I'll think about it."

The lasagna smelled sweet and savory when I pulled it from the oven an hour later. The breadcrumbs on the top were sprinkled with chopped thyme, and the green looked pretty on the creamy goat cheese béchamel. I told Eric about the meeting over dinner.

"Do you think the glasses would help you?" Eric asked Sebastian.

"I don't know," Sebastian replied. He poured his salad dressing on and then replaced the cap. "But the navigation software was interesting."

"They said the navigation software works best with an iPhone," I explained to Eric. I knew Eric wouldn't want to spend the money when he didn't see the necessity, but I tried. "I think we should both upgrade."

"Yeah, your phone's had it," Sebastian agreed. My screen was badly cracked.

"I'll look into it," Eric said, helping himself to another bowl of salad. "This is delicious," he smiled. "It's been a while since you made this."

The compliment didn't conceal what I knew. 'I'll look into it' meant no. Eric wouldn't make a major purchase when he didn't understand the reason. He still didn't understand what was wrong with Sebastian, and I had no idea what else I could say that would convince him when every doctor was telling us that Sebastian was fine. I looked at my plate, suddenly very tired, and poked a bite of lasagna with my fork.

"Once a year, whether you like it or not."

"It's really good, Mom." Sebastian, quicksilver, got it and tried to cheer me up; my heart, my baby, now my almost-grown son. I met his eyes.

"I have an excellent assistant."

***

The neurologist's stare was icy and her posture was stiff as she turned and closed the door after Sebastian's retreating back. Dr. Barb Zegwiller had said little since we had arrived at the appointment, other than to do that thing on the bottom of

Sebastian's feet with the special neurology tool.

The drive into the South Side of Chicago had been surprisingly quick, and the assistant had been friendly and taken excellent notes as I explained the reason for our appointment. I tried to be brief but clear about Sebastian's visual symptoms and how we had discovered them. Sebastian and I had brought his CT scans from the concussion to be reviewed. I was afraid something had been missed. Now, I felt a little unnerved as Dr. Zegwiller's pale brown eyes stared coldly at me.

"He's in a fugue state," she said.

I blinked. I stared at Dr. Zegwiller, thinking, *really? A fugue state? Like some Tom Clancy novel? Is that the best you've got? Does she think I have no wits at all?* A fugue state is a dissociative disorder, the kind with amnesia where some poor soul forgets who they are and wanders around for days or weeks at a time. *What a crock.*

"He's not in a fugue state," I said to the neurologist. "That's ridiculous."

Dr. Zegwiller did not reply but processed to the door and dramatically pulled it open wide. I expected to see her salute as she invited Sebastian back into the room, her short black hair almost militarily erect.

"She said you're in a fugue state," I said as Sebastian walked in. The look on his face was priceless, and if it hadn't been such an awful situation, I think I probably would have laughed.

Sebastian swung around and faced Dr. Zegwiller, who was posed, Statue of Liberty-like, by the desk, her clipboard her lamp of unenlightenment.

"Why did I have to leave the room for that?" Sebastian's voice was rightfully filled with disgust.

Dr. Zegwiller ignored him and launched into her spiel.

"Agnosia is curable with medication," she announced formally. She spoke as though she had her hand on a Bible and was taking an oath. "It is caused by his anxiety, and with anxiety medication his visual memory can be corrected. I have seen it many times."

Instinctively, I knew she was lying. *This is bullshit,* I thought. *Does she think I have no common sense? Or memory?* I was old enough to remember when autism was caused by so-called refrigerator mothers.

I remembered sitting on the scratchy orange shag rug in our family room and watching a documentary on PBS. The old TV with the bunny ear antenna had bad reception, and so the image was somewhat snowy as the little boy spun his plate around and around.

I had never seen a person with autism before. It was in the early 1980s and I was fascinated by this documentary. The narrator explained how in the early days of diagnosis doctors blamed the mother for the condition. They called them "refrigerator mothers" because the theory was that the mothers were so cold and rejecting that the children suffered permanent neurological damage.

Dr. Zegwiller just called me a refrigerator mother, I realized. I felt the heat in my face as I blushed, embarrassed. *Have we learned absolutely nothing over the past fifty years?* My mother's words came back to me. "We believe in science, not religion. We believe in facts that are provable." *What has happened to our medical system?* I wondered.

I knew from Dr. Zegwiller's expression and my own certainty that there wasn't a single credible scientific study anywhere in the world showing that antidepressants cured neurological visual impairments. I sat up taller.

"Sebastian isn't blind because he's anxious," I said flatly. I was polite but no-nonsense. "That's like saying frogs cause warts. He *has* anxiety *because* he's blind, and he's gone for years without necessary orientation and mobility services."

Dr. Zegwiller looked at me like I'd said Sebastian needed anthrax. I forged on anyway.

"He can't recognize environments because he has no visual landmarks, so navigating the way that we do isn't possible for him. I think that most likely he was born this way, and it went undetected because of his extraordinarily high verbal compensation abilities."

Dr. Zegwiller looked nonplussed, but I continued determinedly, and this time cajoling, appealing to her reason. "Sebastian excels at math. He's in AP Calc. Shouldn't he be bad at math with such low visual-spatial scores?" I brandished the neuro psych report. "What does the visual-spatial test measure, if not visual-spatial *abilities*?"

Dr. Zegwiller still did not respond, so I kept on again, this time pleadingly.

"Sebastian doesn't have any academic impairments at all. He's a straight-A honor student. The only assistance he needs is help with navigation. He has environmental agnosia, and he needs a few weeks of orientation and mobility, that's all we're asking for."

Dr. Zegwiller drew herself up ever taller and her pale eyes glared at me. "No. I don't think so."

She said she had to see another patient and turned theatrically to leave. I had to push to get her to review the CT scan from Sebastian's concussion.

"Please, just take a look at it," I pleaded with her. "Maybe something was overlooked."

I handed Dr. Zegwiller Sebastian's CT scan from the concussion in September. She cut her eyes at me in irritation and processed out the door and was gone for several minutes.

Sebastian sat, looking stricken, on the table. *He's not stupid,* I thought. *He knows he just got told he's blind because he's crazy.*

Dr. Zegwiller paraded back through the door and handed me the CD. "It's clear. He can't have agnosia with a normal brain scan. It's impossible. You need to follow up with medication."

Suddenly quick, she disappeared without saying goodbye.

I seethed quietly all the way home. Sebastian was not talking at all. I snuck glances at him with my peripheral vision. I was losing him, and I was tired and angry.

"Why did this have to happen to me?"

"I don't know, honey," I said, tears pricking. "I wish I had an answer for you."

"Brain machine broken."

My jaw dropped, and I put my hand on my heart. "Your brain is not broken. It's everyone else's brains that are," I said, horrified. "You are not defective."

"Yeah. Right."

"You are not," I insisted. "If the world was only half as 'defective' as you are, it would be a much better place. You are the best thing that has ever happened to me. You, and your father."

"Then why is this happening to me?"

"I don't know, sweetie," I said honestly. I rubbed my forehead and pushed my bangs back. I was so exhausted by this whole situation. "I think they just don't have the answers. It's so much easier to just say we're crazy than to try to figure out what's wrong."

"People suck."

"Sometimes they do. Dr. Zegwiller sucks, that's for sure." That didn't bring a smile. "But you don't suck," I said, turning to look at him in the eyes. "You are the bravest person I have ever met in my entire life," I said, realizing as I said the words that it was absolutely true. He walks through this world he can barely perceive visually, and he does everything with grace and beauty, and kindness. He is a miracle.

"I don't feel brave."

"No brave person does. I read somewhere recently about courage. I can't remember all the details, but the article was about ordinary people who did extremely brave things. There was this woman, a preschool teacher, I think." I paused, remembering. "She ran into a burning building and saved a bunch of people, and she was terrified every second she was in there."

Sebastian looked down, frowning, his face a mask of despair. "I don't see what that has to do with me."

"So, the point is, she didn't feel brave. She never felt brave. She just put her head down and ran in."

"So my life is burning down around me."

I sighed. "Pretty much." I paused. "We'll just burn it down together."

Sebastian sat quietly, and then said, "Want to hear a song?"

Peripheral Vision

"The test costs $6,000, whether you test the whole panel of commonly prescribed medications or just the psychotropic drugs," the genetic testing representative said, "so most people choose to test everything. It's a better deal."

Sebastian and I were sitting in the new psychiatrist's office, and we exchanged a look. On the one hand, I was impressed that Dr. Sheltze had arranged for Sebastian's genetic testing on our first meeting. If it was a genetic liver enzyme difference in processing medications that caused Sebastian's bizarre reaction to the Lexapro, we needed to know. On the other hand, $6,000 was a lot of money. The genetic testing rep must have seen my expression, because he immediately leapt in.

"Don't worry, no one ever pays that much. You will get a very scary bill for the six grand. Just ignore it. The genetic testing company has a deal with the insurance companies, but no one ever pays more than $500."

I immediately agreed to run the full panel of genetic testing on Sebastian. I never wanted him to have another drug reaction if I could help it. The last one was frightening enough. I shot a grateful look at Dr. Norm Sheltze, Sebastian's new child psychiatrist. "Thank you so much for having this ready for us."

I was impressed that Dr. Sheltze had the genetic testing representative there at our first meeting. It was Wednesday, February 22, and Dr. Sheltze looked tall and expensive in his designer suit. The attention to his appearance and subtle manscaping stood in sharp contrast to the disorder in his office. Crap was everywhere.

"Serotonin syndrome can be very serious. You must have been quite scared," he replied kindly.

"It was awful," Sebastian said.

Although Dr. Sheltze had been brisk and businesslike with the genetic testing representative, I couldn't help but admire his ability to relate to Sebastian. He really drew him out, and I could see Sebastian trusted him. We talked about Sebastian's vision issues and the history of separation anxiety. He asked if we had a therapist set up, and I told him we had been to see Dr. Bucholz. Dr. Sheltze's handsome face lit up, his blue eyes shining.

"Oh, I'm friends with Drei!" he said.

Cautiously I explained our situation and that Sebastian had scored in the severely impaired range on the diagnostic test for prosopagnosia.

"I'd like to see those test results."

"I requested the face-blindness test results from Dr. Bucholz, but I haven't gotten them yet. I will get them to you once we have them," I assured him. It had been some time since Eric and I faxed the letter to Dr. Bucholz requesting Sebastian's medical records.

When I got home, I called Dr. Bucholz's office and spoke to the receptionist. I politely told her I'd requested Sebastian's records and had not received them.

"I'm so sorry!" the receptionist replied. "I will get those out to you as soon as possible."

I was doubtful. For what felt like the millionth time, I thought about calling a lawyer, but I knew Eric wouldn't agree. He just didn't understand Sebastian's disability, I knew, and he wouldn't spend the money if he didn't see a reason. I didn't know the average attorney's hourly fee, but I knew it was high. I couldn't imagine Eric's reaction to my hiring a lawyer without him, and I couldn't see any scenario where he would agree to one when he wouldn't agree to buy Sebastian an iPhone. I felt alone.

I kept researching and searching agnosia. I read everything I could find, but there was so little information. I checked the website for the National Organization for Rare Diseases. I found the following:

Visual Agnosia

General Discussion

Primary Visual Agnosia is a rare neurological disorder characterized by the total or partial loss of the

> ability to recognize and identify familiar objects and/or people by sight. This occurs without the loss of the ability to actually see the object or person. The symptoms of visual agnosia occur as a result of damage to certain areas of the brain (primary) or in association with other disorders (secondary.)

I continued reading. This condition existed. It was a known thing. I kept reading.

> **Signs and Symptoms**
>
> People with primary visual agnosia may have one or several impairments in visual recognition. Vision is almost always intact and the mind is clear. Some affected individuals do not have the ability to recognize familiar objects. They can see objects but are unable to recognize them by sight. However, objects may be identified by touch, sound, and/or smell. For example, affected individuals may not be able to identify a set of keys by sight, but can identify them by holding them in their hands.

The article on the NORD website went on to describe prosopagnosia (face blindness), object agnosia, and environmental agnosia. It described very closely what I saw in Sebastian's behavior. The thing I noticed that was not stated was that Sebastian recognized words and letters, numbers and simple shapes. Nothing in the article discussed this ability.

I thought, *they do not know. They don't know what we have.* I continued reading.

> **Affected Populations**
>
> Primary visual agnosia is an extremely rare neurological disorder that affects males and females in equal numbers. The first detailed account of visual agnosia in the medical literature occurred in 1890.

Extremely rare, I read again, and the article contained nothing about the ability to use words to recognize things; those two ideas kept me going. This was a known condition, even if it was very rare. I vowed to find someone to help us. My hope lay in the neurology clinic in Southern California. They did cutting-edge research there, my friend had said. There was no better place in the world. *They will help us,* I told myself. They will know. *If only we can get in without a physician referral.* I wondered again what were the odds that they'd see us.

***

I was fuming in the kitchen and chopping my carrots unnecessarily vigorously while I stewed about the low-vision clinic. This low-vision center was just over the border, and though further from other low-vision clinics nearby, it came highly recommended. I'd called them the previous week and the receptionist said the scheduler would call me to set up an appointment by Thursday. When Thursday went by without a peep, I called the out-of-state number again and days later, I'd still had not heard back. I knew I never would.

I finished making dinner and then I quickly folded a load of clean jeans and carried them up the stairs to put away. Sebastian was ironing a shirt in my bedroom.

"Hey. Going somewhere fancy?"

"It's just group tonight."

His smile melted my heart. *He's going to be okay,* I thought.

"Great." I dumped the jeans in a pile to put away later and headed towards the door to go back downstairs. Sebastian turned back to his ironing, all his attention on the task at hand. He was in profile to me, and I could see half his face. It was obvious I was no longer part of his visual awareness.

Something clicked. I remembered a moment from just after we moved to this house. I had folded a basket of laundry. Sebastian was two and a half, or maybe almost three, and he was playing independently in the family room. Rather than disturb his play, I carried the laundry up the stairs and then heard a piercing cry.

"Mama! Mama! Where are you?"

I ran down the stairs, thinking he was hurt. He was fine, but scared. He didn't know where I'd gone. From that point on, I knew, I had made a point of telling him when I was going upstairs. It's a habit we both used to that day. My teenager always told me when he was going to go upstairs, every time, as a courtesy, and I did the same back, not knowing why. It was our normal.

I froze and stared at Sebastian's unnoticing profile. He should have seen me in his peripheral vision, but he was intent on his ironing. It was like I didn't exist.

"I disappear to you, don't I?"

He did not look up.

"Yes."

***

"Did you have a chance yet to look into the iPhones we talked about?" I picked up my water glass and then put it down again. Eric flushed and didn't meet my eyes.

"I haven't had a chance yet."

This is never going to happen, I thought, catching Sebastian's knowing look. Being the sole provider for so many years was stressful for Eric, I knew that. My new Musikgarten business and the small voice studio I ran were gradually making a nice income for me, but my studio was very new and still growing.

I looked more closely at Sebastian's eyes as he sat at the table. There was an odd looseness to the way his eyes were focusing. It was subtle, but there.

"Have you signed up for summer driver's ed yet?" Eric asked Sebastian.

Sebastian looked stricken and shot me a questioning glance.

"Uh, no," Sebastian said carefully. "Was I supposed to? I

didn't think I was doing that."

"I think you probably should," Eric replied, without looking at me.

"He can't," I said. "It's just not safe."

"I think he can," Eric said, still looking at Sebastian. "He can use the Garmin to find his way around."

Sebastian sat, looking from me to his father, his face tense. Eric and I have had very few arguments in twenty-some years of marriage, and while we were not yet arguing, I felt my jaw tighten. How could he not believe his own son? Or me? I squared my shoulders and tried again to explain to Eric why Sebastian couldn't take driver's ed. He needed serious professional safety evaluation and possibly specialized technology, which would require a diagnosis from a doctor.

"No, Eric," I said, looking at him hard. "You don't understand." I thought of Sebastian ironing and not seeing me standing ninety degrees from him. Eric looked at me finally, annoyance on his face.

"I think he can."

"No, he can't," I repeated, my face flushing. Sebastian's stricken eyes looked back at me across the table. My arms prickled as I pictured Sebastian behind the wheel. I took a breath and calmed my tone. "The problem isn't just finding his way around. There are safety concerns with driving. With his visual memory."

"I don't think so," Eric said. "I think he can do it. He might need to use the Garmin to navigate, but he could still drive."

"No!" I said again, thinking of how I disappeared to Sebastian while standing at his side. "Absolutely not." I looked around for something to use as an example, so that Eric could see what I knew. "Look." I took my fork and knife and put them on the table side by side.

"The fork is Sebastian's car," I explained, as I pushed the fork past the knife. When the fork was mostly past the knife, I said, "Once Sebastian can no longer see the car he passes, he has no way of visualizing where that other car is now." Eric looked about to protest, so I rushed ahead. "*You* can." I looked hard at Eric and then pointed at Sebastian. "*He* can't. So, when you pass another car, you can see in your mind approximately how far away the other car is behind you. You can remember its position relative to where you are." I crashed the fork into the knife as though carelessly changing lanes. "He's going to kill someone, and himself, just by changing lanes if you put him behind the wheel. He has no ability to visualize where other cars are around him."

Comprehension bloomed across Eric's face.

"I'm sorry," he admitted. "I finally understand what you've been telling me. I thought it was just a problem with navigating."

Sebastian sagged into his chair in relief, the tension melting out of his face like butter in a warming pan.

"It's okay," Sebastian and I said, together. We laughed with relief, our eyes dancing across the table. We were a family again, and the constant tension in my forehead and shoulders evaporated as I smiled at my two guys. We talked and laughed through dinner, all three of us, and we did not enroll Sebastian in driver's ed.

***

In my continued online research, I found a neuro optometrist and scheduled an appointment for February 27. On their website it said there was treatment for visual memory issues, but all the research I had done indicated that there was no cure for agnosia. I was suspicious but desperate when I called. Dr. Larkin G. Alabaster answered the phone and was very kind. We spoke in depth about what was going on and she asked me to bring in the neuro psych evaluation. We drove all the way to Shorewood for the appointment. Dr. Alabaster was average height and had deep olive skin and lovely, dark mahogany eyes.

After Sebastian's exam, Dr. Alabaster turned to me and said, "Sebastian's condition is curable and we have a treatment plan."

I was doubtful but desperate at this point. Even if the treatment is only slightly successful, I reasoned, it would be better than nothing.

"You can fix his gaze?" I asked, looking up at this kindly woman. Dr. Alabaster's deep brown eyes looked back at me with sympathy. "I can tell just from looking at his face that his eyes are too loosely focused. It's subtle, but it's there."

"We can fix that too," she said confidently, but she didn't tell me more, or what Sebastian's eye-tracking condition was called. "Vision therapy isn't usually covered by insurance," Dr. Alabaster said. "It's $150 a session. After ten sessions we'll reassess."

I talked it over with Eric later.

"That's a lot of money," he said. "I think we should wait."

Frustrated and completely forgetting our breakthrough in understanding Sebastian's vision impairment at dinner just days before, I felt unsupported at every turn.

I cried, "Wait for what? If there's any possibility his vision can be fixed, I'm taking it. I'm signing him up."

***

This guy is wonderful, I thought, as I watched Dr. Sheltze talking with Sebastian. It was February 28 and it was Sebastian's second appointment with this new psychiatrist. Dr. Shelze really drew Sebastian out. No wonder he had such a busy practice. Sebastian was laughing and telling him all about the school arts fair coming up.

We received the report from the genetic testing company. Sebastian did indeed have a genetic liver enzyme deficiency or difference in processing medications. Then we discussed Sebastian's progress at the anxiety day program. Sebastian was doing really well with the anxiety management techniques, but we were both relieved when Dr. Sheltze prescribed Sebastian Pristiq before we left.

***

On March 3, Sebastian began vision therapy with Dr.

Alabaster, once a week for ten weeks.

***

"Why don't you bring in the report," the pharmacist said kindly to me on the phone. "Let me take a look at it."

I sagged with relief. Sebastian was having unusual bleeding, a potentially serious side effect of Pristiq. Since these things never happen during business hours, I had to have Dr. Sheltze paged on a weekend afternoon. He had told me to call the pharmacy and have them check for possible drug interactions with Sebastian's one other prescription, and I couldn't make either heads or tails of this report from the genetic testing lab.

Sebastian and I arrived at the pharmacy ten minutes later, and my concern rose as the pharmacist spent the next thirty minutes checking various websites and making phone calls before he could tell us if Pristiq had drug interactions with the one other medication my son was on. I thanked the pharmacist profusely for taking so much time to help us out, and we shook hands. He waved off the compliment. "Of course. It's my job."

As Sebastian and I turned to leave, the pharmacist called after us. "For medical safety reasons you should ask the prescriber for the list of commonly prescribed medications that are safe for Sebastian. This list only includes psychotropic medications."

We requested the whole panel.

I picked up Sebastian from his group at church at nine just a couple of days later. It was the first week of March, and Sebastian said he wasn't feeling well. It was after nine o'clock at night and he said he felt super wide awake, uncomfortable, and that everything felt abnormally hilarious. He did not look well.

At home I checked the side effects for Pristiq, and mania was a dangerous one. I followed the directions and called Dr. Sheltze immediately. It was about 9:30 p.m. The answering service paged Dr. Sheltze, and he returned my call swiftly, to my great relief. I thanked him for his caring response and briefly explained the situation.

"You need to reduce his dosage of Pristiq," Dr. Sheltze said, and "because the pills aren't scored, there is no safe way to cut them in half." For that reason, he said, "Sebastian should take one pill every other day." We immediately followed Dr. Sheltze's directions and Sebastian's symptoms were better the next day.

On Friday, March 17, we had Sebastian's third appointment with Dr. Sheltze. When I picked up Sebastian from school, he was feeling positive about being back in school part time. He had a very good day in art and with his friends. Spending time with April at lunch had really lifted his spirits. We were both relaxed and happy and had a cheerful discussion about his experiences that day on our way to the appointment.

As we walked into the reception area, I noticed that the normally busy waiting area was empty. The messy-haired, black eye-linered receptionist took our names and then immediately disappeared.

Dr. Sheltze opened the door and walked us back to his office, looking elegant in his tailored suit and green-striped St. Patrick's Day tie.

"Things are going really well with Sebastian's return to school," I said as I sat on that luscious sofa. "The pharmacist double-checked and there are no known drug interactions with the other medication, and the bleeding has stopped. I think we're good."

Dr. Sheltze listened professionally and took notes.

"Oh," I remembered, "the pharmacist recommended that we get the list of safe, commonly prescribed medications for Sebastian today. We only got the report for psychotropic drugs."

The change in Dr. Sheltze's appearance and demeanor was sudden and dramatic. His eyes flashed and he changed the subject.

"Where is your medication?" he asked Sebastian.

Sebastian glanced at me and looked back at Dr. Sheltze. He shook his head. "I didn't bring it."

Dr. Sheltze's face contorted and he turned to me angrily.

"Why didn't you bring his medication with you in a plastic bag?"

I blinked, surprised. "This is the first I have ever heard of having to bring medications," I said calmly. "I didn't know we were supposed to."

Dr. Sheltze exploded, hunting through the piles on his desk and on the shelves behind him, raging. He lifted up files and books and looked under a pile of papers. Then he shouted at Sebastian, "How am I supposed to know what medication you are taking, and what the dosage is?"

I sat frozen in shock as Dr. Sheltze resumed rummaging through the piles of papers everywhere. I couldn't even formulate a thought, let alone a reply. He saw the look on my face and stopped digging.

"How are you cutting the pills?" Dr. Sheltze shouted.

With as much dignity and courtesy as I could manage, which was a lot, I calmly replied, "We aren't cutting the pills. You told us not to because they aren't scored, and you said there was no safe way to cut them." Dr. Sheltze's face contorted as I finished speaking. "You told us to reduce his dosage by going to one pill every other day. The pharmacist told us to get the list for the commonly prescribed medications. We need it for safety reasons."

Dr. Sheltze became verbally and emotionally abusive towards me. I have never seen anybody act like this, except my mother.

"You had no business taking that report all over town," he snarled. "Your anxiety is ridiculous," he continued, throwing papers all over his desk.

I sat there, staring. To my readers, I want to assure you that this is not a work of fiction: I was appalled at this doctor's behavior, and shocked. That report was our property. What we did with it was our business. This crazy psychiatrist was attacking me for following his own instructions. I goggled at him, wordless.

"You should just *take a weekend* or something," Dr. Sheltze snapped rudely.

The only person in the room who needed some time off was

Dr. Sheltze. Sebastian and I exchanged an appalled look, envisioning Dr. Sheltze on a nice, long vacation, in a padded room with a special white jacket. I turned my attention silently back to the doctor. He was ransacking his piles and yelling. Sebastian sat frozen next to me, silent.

We got up and we left.

"Have a good day," I managed. I cried in the car in the parking lot.

Over dinner I tried to talk about what happened with Eric. Sebastian's therapist and his vision therapy put our monthly medical bills at over $1,000 a month. Eric shrugged unhappily.

"We really can't afford a lawyer," he said. "I really think you should just find another doctor."

We had to find another psychiatrist to fill Sebastian's Pristiq prescription. Sebastian and I were both emotionally devastated and exhausted. This would be our third psychiatrist. I was more than aware of how this looked. My mother was a doctor shopper. She'd just shop around until she could find the one who would tell her what she wanted to hear.

I had several friends who were nurses. I asked around and got another name for a very highly regarded child psychiatrist. We would have to travel out of state to see him, but it was only a couple of hours away. I made an appointment with Sebastian for the eighteenth of April. I was afraid.

Satyr with Mask

"I stood transfixed, listening... and knew what can never be expressed: that the natural is supernatural, and that I am the eye that hears and the ear that sees, that what is outside happens in me, that outside and inside are unseparated." - Frederick Franck

I hung up the phone, my heart surging with hope. Char Laursen, our new speech pathologist, had worked with students with agnosias before. I couldn't believe it. Char had been wonderful and engaging on the phone and told me she'd be checking Sebastian for anomia, an inability to retrieve words. I laughed, and then told her Sebastian wrote a novel back in middle school.

"We'd have noticed if he'd had anomia," I explained, but I agreed we should follow our audiologist's recommendations to see her. I made the appointment for the speech evaluation. I didn't know if there was anything else we had missed, as the vision impairment had gone undetected. Maybe there were other issues we didn't know of yet.

Char Laursen was genuine, friendly, and kind. Her cheerful face was sweet, and she was clearly intrigued by Sebastian. It was March 21 and we were there to begin the first portion of the speech assessment on Sebastian. Not unexpectedly, he sailed through it, as we knew he would. Char treated us like we were normal people, without a hint of skepticism or doubt. I was filled with renewed hope and optimism just because Char treated us like human beings deserving of respect and assistance. I had forgotten what that was like.

A few days later, after his vision therapy appointment with Dr. Alabaster, Sebastian told me he hated vision therapy and that he spent most of his time crossing and uncrossing his eyes. I told him to bear with it in case it actually helped in some way. Sebastian told me his vision was not changing, and neither was the weird looseness to his focus that I could see. I was getting absolutely no information about Sebastian's condition or his progress from Dr. Alabaster.

"We'll discuss everything after the ten-week assessment. It's too early to say now," Dr. Alabaster said, her deep brown eyes crinkling reassuringly. I was not reassured.

Sebastian got one vision therapy activity to work on at home after the first session, but nothing was given after that.

***

"Look! He has a bird draped across his shoulders!" Sebastian said.

It was spring break and we were exploring early Greek and Roman art at the Art Institute of Chicago when we found our totem. His name was Striding Figure and I was smitten in a way I have never experienced before. Striding Figure was a Proto-Elamite or Mesopotamian copper alloy sculpture. He was about five thousand years old, and Sebastian and I were entranced.

"He's beautiful," I breathed.

The wings of some large bird of prey were draped across the tiny sculpture's muscular shoulders, and the body of the bird hung down the man's back. The horns of an ibex, which curved back from his headgear, rose upwards from his head, and a pointed beard graced his lovely face. His upturned boots were elfin and reminiscent of short skis.

Striding Figure's arms and legs were poised in the middle of a step, but it was his eyes that fascinated me. His white shell eyes turned humbly up to the heavens. He was not demanding or threatening. He was humbly asking, for what I was not sure. Sebastian and I couldn't take our eyes off the tiny ancient sculpture.

"Look," Sebastian pointed. "His left hand was curled to hold something, but whatever was there is gone. What do you think he was holding?" Sebastian asked, his eyes shining with curiosity.

"I was just wondering the same thing myself. An umbrella?"

I quirked my eyebrow at Sebastian.

Sebastian laughed. “A badminton racquet?”

“A fly swatter?” I was in full swing now. “Maybe a bunch of balloons.”

We were standing in the quiet museum and I was cackling with laugher. People were giving us looks. *Maybe we really are crazy,* I thought, hilariously. I was in love with this little statue. During our tour of the museum we also discovered Satyr with Mask.

“Hey, Sebastian. Check this out! This huge bearded mask is a Greek theater mask of Silenos.”

“Maybe he’ll bless your coq au vin.”

Sebastian and I circled around the bizarre sculpture. The mask itself was the bearded and frightening face of an angry adult man, with holes for the eyes and mouth. The satyr’s tiny toddler hand protruded from the angry mouth, like a baby traffic officer commanding us to stop and see. I obeyed the command willingly.

Little chubby toddler legs emerged from underneath the massive mask, and a sweet little hand held the mask up. I was enchanted by the playful satyr peeking out through the eyes of the frightful mask. I knew the feeling of trying to see through someone else’s eyes.

I was beginning to think people were so terrified of being blind that they couldn’t even begin to imagine what Sebastian’s vision was like because they didn’t want to. They were too afraid. I vividly remembered my own terror at first discovering Sebastian’s agnosias. The idea of having nothing and no one ever look familiar made me feel like I was falling off the world, as though I were the one who was, again, lost.

After our tour of the museum, Sebastian and I walked the few blocks around the Art Institute. As we walked the busy city streets, Sebastian’s difficulty navigating became more and more apparent. I asked Sebastian if he knew how to get back to the museum. It was only a block away and we had just walked by it. He had no idea. His confusion was completely obvious in an unfamiliar environment. Even though I expected to see some difficulty navigating, the seriousness of Sebastian's disability was overwhelming.

"I have been a goat, or pony, I realized just now," I said to him. "You know, even barnyard animals lead their blind friends around the pasture." I wondered if they knew their friend was blind, or if they just sensed the other animal was anxious when they strayed too far away. I guessed it was the second, and was struck again at how many humans refuse to recognize that animals feel emotions like compassion. "I've seen it on the news. We've all been leading you, without knowing it."

"I'm really good at following, too," Sebastian admitted. "I can follow you even when you are behind me."

He stepped in front and to the side of me, and using his peripheral motion vision, he kept pace with me. Just like his inexplicable eye contact from his earliest days as a baby masked his face blindness, his ability to follow from the front masked his inability to navigate.

Before we went home that afternoon, Sebastian and I practiced his routes between the dorm where he would be staying for his oil painting class in June and the entrance to his class building at the School of the Art Institute. We walked the short three- or four-block pattern several times. At the end, Sebastian still had no idea where anything was.

Worse still, several times he walked out into traffic following a jaywalker. I had to yank him back onto the sidewalk by his arm. He missed getting hit by a car by inches. Living on an extremely quiet street in a very small and sleepy neighborhood concealed a lot from us. The blinders kept coming off my eyes, little by little.

I had never seen Sebastian step into traffic before, ever, but I of course had a memory. April told me once that she saved him from getting hit while they were out together downtown. She had seen him step right into traffic and done the Costanza "stop short."

***

Nothing was changing with Sebastian's vision therapy. I received zero feedback from Dr. Alabaster on what his diagnosis was, what the prognosis was, or what he should be practicing at home. Every time I asked, I was stonewalled.

"Don't worry, we'll go over everything with you at the ten-week progress report. It's too early yet to evaluate his progress," she said, brown eyes warm and kind.

***

The warm scent of homemade pasta and sauces filled the dining room as I found my way back to our table at Clara's Italian restaurant. It was March 27, and I hadn't seen some of these friends since high school; I was eager to reconnect. I wound my way through the tables to find my friends. Patty Kelly, who had been so comforting and helpful when I first discovered Sebastian's vision impairment, was waiting.

It was exciting to see friends I hadn't seen in decades, and we all hugged. Tish Calhamer, who had attended the University of Illinois with me after high school, was now the community engagement officer at the Gail Borden Library in Elgin. My lovely friend Julie K. Jessen, an accomplished wildlife photographer and travel specialist, and her husband, Cliff Passmore, joined us as well. Dear friends Sue Czechowicz and Carol Reinheimer completed our group.

We shared a bottle of cabernet. I was that friend at the high school reunion who talked for the entire meal, nonstop. Tish tells me I was saying things like, "I must be the worst mother in the whole world! How could I not see that something was terribly wrong with my own child?"

Tish says she told me, "The usual signs that something is wrong with your kid are failing classes, slumping grades, belligerent behavior, that kind of thing. Sebastian was bringing home A-pluses! He got the lead in the church musical! He excelled at the Young Entrepreneurs Academy. You couldn't have known something was wrong in the middle of all that achievement."

Tish tells me I was laughing and crying at that point.

I told the entire story. Everything. No one called me crazy or told me Sebastian would get better with anti-anxiety medications. Maybe no one got a word in edgewise, but still, no one had to leave early. I told everyone about Dr. Bucholz and Dr. Sturgis dropping us from their care without a referral. The story just poured out of me.

"Dr. Bucholz said they were dropping us for quote, unquote 'Legal and ethical reasons.' He said Sebastian shouldn't have received visual memory testing so soon after having his visual-spatial testing for the concussion," I marveled. "Can you believe these doctors? They acted like we're going to sue them over a clerical error, and all we did was thank them kindly."

"That's ridiculous," Patty said. "When we see errors like this in OT, it just means that you take the test results with a grain of salt."

I remember the sense of shock sitting there at the table. All this time I had been flabbergasted at being dropped from Dr. Bucholz's care, and so confused about the reason why. I realized I probably never would know the exact reason Dr. Bucholz dropped us. My guess was that Dr. Bucholz was embarrassed to be wrong about the Effexor being safe for Sebastian. Effexor is not a non-serotonin medication, as he'd claimed.

Sitting there in the restaurant, I realized for the first time that Dr. Bucholz probably decided to label us as crazy rather than admit to his own medical mistake. I did know that leaving us in a crisis without even a referral to another psychologist was unethical. All these months we had been bouncing from doctor to doctor without the one piece of evidence that would show that my son had a problem: the prosopagnosia face-blindness test results. Dr. Bucholz set us up to look like we were nuts.

I could hear the crazy psychiatrist, the handsome huckster Dr. Sheltze's voice, "Oh, I'm friends with Drei!"

Dr. Bucholz and Dr. Sheltze had talked. I was certain there

was illegal and unethical communication going on between these doctors regarding us. I remembered something else, too. I could still see the messy-haired receptionist with the black eyeliner, who had dodged away so abruptly after taking our names at our last appointment with Dr. Sheltze. I remembered glancing behind her to see if someone else was there; she had appeared that visibly frightened.

I remember briefly thinking she might be in danger, and feeling a vague surprise, concern, and confusion, until I realized we were alone in the normally busy waiting room. It was such a strange and memorable interaction. I guessed now that the receptionist knew Dr. Sheltze had it in for us, and the waiting room was empty because she had canceled all of Dr. Sheltze's afternoon appointments so there'd be no witnesses to the shouting.

On the way home, I realized another thing: I was coming down with a sinus infection. I was grieving for Dr. Fredericks. Is it weird to grieve your own doctor? I felt like I'd lost part of my family. I grieved for the doctor I'd trusted for a quarter of a century.

***

A few days later my phone rang.

"Hello?" I said automatically. I knew who it was, but I couldn't believe it.

Lukas's warm baritone was friendly and calm. He said he was flying into the area for a conference in mid-April and he asked if we'd like to have dinner. I have no words for what I felt. Imagine drowning for four solid months. You keep almost going under, and yet for some reason you're not dead yet.

I made a reservation at Meson Sabika, our favorite Spanish tapas restaurant.

Lukas's brilliance was not at all hidden behind a very modest and unassuming facade. He was extremely intelligent, and that intense perceptiveness was immediately apparent. We ordered tapas and made conversation. Lukas worked with the deaf-blind; he taught people who had deaf-blindness to get around using a guide dog. He shared a few fascinating stories of some of his experiences.

Lukas was interested in Sebastian's art ability. He asked to see some of Sebastian's art, and they talked about it. He told us his father had passed away a few years back. He said his father wrote an art book called *The Zen of Seeing: Seeing/Drawing as Meditation.* Eric purchased the book off Amazon at the table. Lukas kindly turned the conversation to how Sebastian navigated. Sebastian explained that he counted his steps and turns everywhere he went.

"How would you find the bathroom?" Lukas asked.

"I can see the sign from here," Sebastian said. "I would count my steps and turns to the sign and figure it out from there by the signs on the bathroom doors. Then I just reverse it to get back."

Lukas asked Sebastian if he ever used physical objects to navigate. He asked Sebastian if he had his back to a rock, could he walk forward until he came to another object, like a bench? He put the concepts together, rock/bench.

Sebastian didn't know. He had never tried to navigate in that manner, and it was frightening and confusing for him.

Lukas took Sebastian around the restaurant and had him try different things, such as putting his back to the hostess stand and using that physical landmark as a starting point for navigation. Sebastian tried it, but clearly had his own way of doing things and was unnerved by trying to change so suddenly. Then with our permission, Lukas took Sebastian out to the parking lot to try navigating outside. We talked about it when they both returned.

Sebastian had never considered using the rock/bench physical object mode of navigation and I could tell it scared him to try something different. He had taught himself his own way of counting steps and turns. He had no experience with any other way. It was obvious Lukas could see that Sebastian's mode of navigation was not typical for a sighted person, and I felt hugely validated that someone else could see what I saw.

Because Sebastian had no academic impairments, I told Lukas I didn't think we could get an IEP through the school, since schools don't usually just hand out IEPs to their top students. Without an IEP, I was pretty sure we'd have difficulty getting O&M training through the school. Lukas told us he would try to help us find a private O&M instructor for Sebastian in case we couldn't get help through the school.

We were overwhelmed with gratitude. Lukas gave Sebastian his card and invited him to contact him after he had had a chance to practice some of the new techniques. We took a picture of Sebastian and Lukas before he left.

A day or two later, a package arrived. I opened it eagerly, and found a book: *The Zen of Seeing: Seeing/Drawing as Meditation.* It had a yellow cover and was all beautifully handwritten and illustrated by the artist, Frederick Franck. My curiosity piqued, I Googled him and found his page on Wikipedia. In his humility, Lukas did not tell us his father was a famous artist and a prolific author.

I read, fascinated. Frederick Franck was a western Zen master, and an extraordinary artist with works in many major museums. He had devoted his life to peace on earth and had created a beautiful sculpture garden at his home in Warwick, New York. He called it Pacem in Terris.

I eagerly turned to my new book, and I was immediately drawn into the story of how Frederick Franck was invited to teach a drawing course. The older Franck entitled this chapter "An Experiment in Seeing That Became 'An Unforgettable Experience.'" Lukas's father described how he took on the not-much-desired task of teaching a course entitled "Creativity in a Non-Creative Environment." *More people need to read this book,* I thought, as I admired the mind behind the beautiful words, the precise calligraphy, and the delicate drawings.

I read, fascinated, and there it was on page four: the answer I had been looking for since January, found in an art book written by the famous artist father of a brilliant orientation and mobility specialist. The key to how Sebastian could see while blind, and why he is a gifted artist, was in Frederick Franck's book. Frederick Franck stated:

> "We do a lot of looking: we look through lenses, telescopes, television tubes... Our looking is perfected every day - but we see less and less. Never has it been more urgent to speak of SEEING. Ever more gadgets, from cameras to computers, from art books to video tapes, conspire to take over our thinking, our feeling, our experiencing, our seeing. Onlookers we are, spectators... "Subjects" we are, that look at "Objects." Quickly we stick labels on all that is, labels that stick once- and for all. By these labels we recognize everything- but no longer SEE anything. We know the labels on all the bottles, but never taste the wine."

I sat back on the sofa. I saw how my son sees. I had seen his blindness, his vision without recognition. I knew his imperception of anything except symbols. I saw O G D E N A V E in that maelstrom of unrecognizable chaos. Now, my blinders were again removed. I saw my son's visual perception.

Sebastian's labels didn't attach. He had to attach a label, a word, to see things. He didn't just see words; he saw *WITH* words.

I sat there, in wonder. Was it possible? Could it be true? I knew for a fact that my son saw with a newborn's eyes; a newborn who could read, I corrected myself. Could he be labeling every single object and person and animal with characteristics, characteristics that must be reattached, every single time? And getting a visual image, not just guessing an answer? Could he literally see with words the way a bat sees with sound?

Sebastian must be getting a visual image with his inner narration, I decided. How else could anyone explain the speed of his visual processing, which was so fast he appeared to be typically sighted? I asked him.

"I don't know," he said. "But nothing ever looks familiar to me except words, letters, numbers, and simple shapes."

***

In April, Lukas called and connected me to a local well-known, retired O&M specialist. He and Gala Brooks were both trying to help us to find a local O&M specialist. I spoke with Gala, who was so helpful and kind. I told her I was offering $100 an hour for a private O&M instructor. She was enjoying travel in her retirement, and she cheerfully agreed to search for someone local with the skills to help Sebastian.

It was official, but not a surprise, when a day or two later, Char Laursen told us Sebastian did not have anomia. It was April 17, our last speech assessment, and Sebastian sailed through the test. Word retrieval was not a problem for Sebastian. He was the king of le mot juste.

Sebastian aced the final speech assessment, and out of boredom went on to correct the punctuation and spelling errors embedded in the test, to my amusement. Afterwards, Char went over the scores and noticed that Sebastian got one item wrong. Sebastian mistakenly labeled a backhoe as a dump truck.

In my experience, many people of lesser perception would have seized on this moment of imperfection to exult in Sebastian's error; they would thrill to find a visible sign that he was not as intelligent as he actually is. Char did not. Instead, with her typical acumen, Char asked Sebastian how he arrived at this one incorrect answer. I could have kissed her. Her insight gave me the key to Sebastian's visual processing that we'd been missing.

Thoughtfully considering her question about the backhoe, Sebastian answered: "Well, first I knew it was a 'thing.' Then I knew it was a 'vehicle' because of the wheels/treads," he explained. "Then I knew it was a construction vehicle because it was yellow, but I didn't know what the digger on the end was, so I labeled it a bulldozer. That was as close as I could get to figuring it out."

Sebastian was using a taxonomy of verbal characteristics to identify objects. Although I believed him when he told me he could recognize only symbols and simple shapes, I needed some other evidence to believe he also had object agnosia, to truly come to grips with the scale of Sebastian's semantic memory.

I asked him, "Do you do this for everything? Build one characteristic on top of another in a taxonomy?"

Sebastian didn't pause. "Everything starts off as a thing," he said simply. He considered the question more carefully. "You know what's interesting?"

"What?" Char and I watched him, fascinated to see what he would say next.

"A backhoe and a goose are like synonyms: they both have long necks with a pointy thing on the end." Then he had another thought. "A measuring spoon and an igloo are also like synonyms: a round dome with a projection on it."

Up until this point, Sebastian's use of sublingual vocalization (silent narration) to see had been almost entirely unconscious to him. His visual processing appeared to be as fast as neurotypical visual processing, except in the case of moving objects, like traffic. The constant subconscious stream of words he used to see were too fast for him to notice until it was slowed down in this simple exercise. Char's simple and perceptive question solved the uncertainty; Sebastian had object agnosia.

Char, Sebastian, and I had a long conversation about this new discovery about Sebastian's verbal visual processing. Together we discussed Sebastian's ability to recognize his environment. He had none. Char agreed with me that Sebastian needed a referral for occupational therapy for navigation. As a speech pathologist, she said, she couldn't write one for us. She suggested we ask our neurologist to write the prescription for OT.

I didn't want to bad-mouth a doctor in front of Char, so I said nothing to Char about Dr. Zegwiller and the ridiculous "fugue state" diagnosis. When I got home, I called Dr. Zegwiller's office and left a message, explaining that Char Laursen told us Sebastian needed a referral for OT for navigation. I got a call back. Dr. Zegwiller refused to provide the referral. I was not surprised.

I had no choice. I called Dr. Fredericks's office and left a message explaining what was needed and why. Not long after, I received a phone call. I recognized this person's voice. I had had many polite and cordial conversations with her over the years. This person was sarcastic, rude, and brutal. There were no pleasantries.

"Do you even know why he needs this?" she snarled.

All the Same Channels

I tried to breathe. This woman's open hostility and rudeness slapped my face through the phone. I had had it, and months of frustration and anger boiled up.

"Because he's blind!" I shouted. "Aaargh!"

Yes, I really did make the "Aaargh!" noise while I punched the hang-up button. I didn't include it in what eventually turned into my thirty-six single-spaced typed pages of documentation of what a shit-show our lives had become. I just remember the tear on my vocal folds and the fact that I held my phone away from me while I aarghed directly at it.

As I was sitting in the kitchen lamenting that an entire generation had grown up without knowing the thrill of slamming a handset down, it occurred to me that during this entire journey, I had been unpleasant to a medical professional once. This was the first time I had been rude to anyone. It felt awesome.

Dr. Fredericks's office made the referral for occupational therapy.

***

"I'd like to add a neuropsychologist to the team, if that's okay with you." Dr. Kakalec was extremely professional, despite the man-bun and wrinkled shirt, and I felt a rush of relief as his compassion and concern radiated across the table.

"That's wonderful," I said, "I think he needs a team."

I looked with gratitude at our new psychiatrist and felt some of the tension of the past months release. Sebastian and I were both tired from our hours-long drive out of state to this appointment, but we needed a psychiatrist who would fill Sebastian's prescription for Pristiq. Dr. Kakalec had been very warm and obviously concerned as we filled him in on all we had discovered.

I was hopeful that the promised neuropsychologist would be

able to diagnose Sebastian's vision impairment and we could go on with our lives. We had no time left for questions, though, because the hour had been spent on Sebastian's exhaustive medical history and how we had discovered everything. Sebastian was smiling when we said goodbye to Dr. Kakalec. There were friendly handshakes all around. The appointment ended cordially, and I scheduled the next two visits with the receptionist before we left.

Later that afternoon I sat in agony. *Should I tell the handsome fraudster Dr. Sheltze that I had changed Sebastian to this new psychiatrist? For continuity of care, what should I do?* We had another appointment with Dr. Sheltze still on the books that I needed to cancel. I had never received the full genetic testing panel I paid for. I had called several times.

I researched lawyers and looked for a low-cost one, but on paper we wouldn't quality for assistance. We were drowning in medical bills. Sebastian's new therapist was wonderful, totally on board with his vision impairment and everything, but she wasn't on our insurance plan. Between the audiologist, the vision therapy, speech therapy assessments, and Sebastian's psychologist, our monthly costs had metastasized.

I slowly picked up the phone and left a polite message.

"Hello, this message is for Dr. Sheltze. This is Stephanie Duesing calling for my son, Sebastian. We will not be at his next appointment. We are changing to a different doctor for personal reasons. We still have not received the full panel of genetic testing that we paid for. We need to have that before our next appointment."

***

"What is that?" The occupational therapist pointed at the gigantic Connect Four game and then looked at Sebastian.

It was April 24, 2017, and it was about to be a very big day in our lives. Our OT assessor had taken Sebastian all around the large, equipment-filled room and asked him to identify different objects as we walked: chairs, tables, a toddler jungle gym. Now, we were standing at the center of the room looking at a three-foot-tall version of the Connect Four game. I could picture ours at home underneath Monopoly in the basement closet. I wanted to shout the answer to Sebastian, but I just stood and watched.

Silence.

I could see the wheels turning in Sebastian's head and I watched in amazement as he pondered. We played Connect Four often when Sebastian was little. He knew this game. Sebastian was still standing there, flummoxed. I started counting the seconds. It took Sebastian more than ten seconds to identify the game, and then only after he picked up a disk, inserted it into the slot, and watched it hit the bottom of the track.

"It's a Connect Four game," Sebastian said, his eyebrows raised high, his eyes wide with wonder. "I couldn't recognize it because it doesn't match my characteristics. Ours at home is small."

This moment on April 24, 2017 was the first time in my life that I had ever seen my son struggle to recognize an object. He was fifteen years old.

"What about it made it hard for you to identify?" the OT asked him, perceptively.

"It was too big," Sebastian said, "and so I couldn't recognize it. It didn't match my characteristics."

The OT recommended that we come three days a week to work on navigation. I was exultant. We scheduled appointments for Monday, Tuesday, and Wednesday afternoons with the wonderful and kind Kaitlyn Peters. I did not document these appointments because there was no need. We went religiously to every single one.

At occupational therapy Kaitlyn helped Sebastian to get a Ventra card and taught him how to use Google Maps to navigate Chicago. Kaitlyn clearly wasn't sure what was wrong with Sebastian, but she knew how to teach people with visual impairments how to get around. She was friendly and kind to both of us. We liked and respected her greatly.

She taught Sebastian how to navigate on foot, using Google Maps. Then he learned the city bus system, the subway, and the El. He learned to use Uber and Lyft. Taxis were harder, because they had to be flagged down and he had difficulty seeing them coming. I was grateful we lived in the twenty-first century and had cell phones.

Sebastian and I went three times a week into Chicago for occupational therapy through the first week of August. From April 24 until Sebastian left for his oil painting class on June 18, we practiced his routes around the School of the Art Institute campus on those trips into the city. I parked in the parking garage at the OT center, and either before or after his appointment, Sebastian was responsible for taking me on public transit over to the museum campus. We practiced his routes three times per week to get him ready to live in the dorms that summer.

With the practice, we both lost our intense fear of getting lost. Having a Garmin changed our lives, because we knew it would always get us home.

On April 25 at 9:00 a.m. we had our second appointment with Dr. Kakalec, our third child psychiatrist. Sebastian and I left early again to make it across state lines in time. We were both tired when we arrived. We walked down the hall to Dr. Kakalec's office together and I opened the door. The doctor glared angrily at me as I opened the door.

I shied back, confused by the overt hostility in the man's eyes. I glanced quickly around the room and saw that the promised neuropsychologist was not there. Dr. Kakalec was extremely unfriendly and rude to me, in front of Sebastian, for the entire appointment. When I asked if he would refill Sebastian's prescription for Pristiq, he said nastily that he "was not treating him, only assessing him." He said, for the first time, that "the decision to accept him as a patient won't be made until after the third appointment on June 6."

I was stunned, embarrassed, and totally humiliated. I was scared for Sebastian's safety. I had no one now to fill Sebastian's anxiety medication. Sebastian went completely white beside me. He was silent and visibly afraid.

I politely apologized and explained to Dr. Kakalec that I wasn't told that Sebastian was not his patient yet. Dr. Kakalec adjusted his man-bun and coldly said that the person who originally scheduled our appointment should have told me. I politely explained again that this was the first time I'd heard of this policy. Dr. Kakalec was openly rude and dismissive of my concerns for Sebastian's mental health and safety.

The entire meeting was hostile and awkward. There was a palpable sense of disbelief. We left shortly afterwards, totally embarrassed. I don't think either Sebastian or I said a word on the long ride home from out of state.

In the car on the way home from school a few days later, Sebastian told me he hated vision therapy, again.

"Dr. Alabaster has me do this thing where I walk on the balance beam," Sebastian said. "I'm supposed to say the alphabet backwards while I do it."

"And?" I asked. Sebastian hadn't talked much about what goes on during his vision therapy session, except to say he hated it. I had been unsuccessful in drawing him out. I tried again. "What happens?"

"There's this arrow projected on the wall," Sebastian explained. "It changes direction, and I'm supposed to use this clicker thing to show what direction it's pointing while I walk the balance beam." He paused, thinking, unsure if he should continue.

I was listening carefully, wondering where this was going.

"And?" I prompted. I didn't want him to clam up. "What happens then?"

Sebastian hesitated, uncomfortable. Then finally it came out in a rush. "When I am doing it," he said. "I mean, when I am walking on the balance beam and saying the alphabet backwards at the same time," he paused again. "I can't see the arrow at all. I can't see anything."

I didn't know how to process this, so I just sat there.

Sebastian was genuinely disturbed. I was, too. I exhaled and shook my head, unable to find words to respond. Finally, I turned to him. His eyes were like holes.

"I hate going, Mom," he said again.

Guilt suffused me. What had I done?

"I feel like Dr. Alabaster thinks I could see if I would just try harder."

My heart was breaking for my son, again, for, what, the millionth time since January? How many times can your heart break before you just give up?

"I will never give up until we get you some help," I promised him. "Nothing can make me stop."

He looked at me, then looked away, his face tight.

"No matter how far we slide backwards, nothing and no one can ever make me stop."

I was crying now for him, for all the years of fear and sorrow, and all the ignorance and fear he was facing so graciously from so-called medical professionals who, one after another, had no qualms about hurting a child; a child who needed only the most basic, small help. We weren't asking for controlled substances or unneeded surgery. I was furious for my child. I was exhausted, and I was scared.

At home, I had to dismantle my Musikgarten business because the OT in the afternoons and all the doctor appointments conflicted with my teaching schedule. I refunded all my families' tuition. Any last hopes of hiring a lawyer went out the door with the checks. We finished the church musical the week before occupational therapy started, so I didn't have to worry about my Wednesday Cherubim Choir rehearsals, at least. My sweet little ones and I had our pizza party and we were done for the season. At our last Musikgarten classes, we took photos, and sweet mamas brought small gifts.

"Let us know when you're ready. We'll come back," they promised.

"Thanks," I replied, feeling genuinely touched. "This is hard."

"Don't worry about it," one mom smiled at me. "When you

go to California, they will help you. My dad went, and they will have a team ready for you when you arrive. It's amazing."

I felt tears pricking my eyes at her kindness and relief that we'd been accepted at the neurology clinic without a physician referral. I ducked my head.

"We have an appointment with a neuro ophthalmologist coming up. Should I cancel?" I asked her. "We've been waiting almost four months for this appointment."

"Don't cancel," she assured me. "The neurologists in California will be glad for his report when you go."

I gave her a little smile, and she hugged me again. "It will be okay. They were amazing with my father, and they'll take good care of you."

***

The following week, on April 25, we were seated in a new pediatrician's office, and I was pressing my lips together and trying to look polite.

"Hmmm... Let's see," Dr. Shah said, theatrically.

Dr. Shah was short and round, and her beautiful green-flecked hazel eyes sparked unpleasantly at me as she pulled up a chart on her computer. It was the week after our disaster with Dr. Kakalec and his man-bun. Sebastian needed his Pristiq prescription filled. He was almost out. We had nowhere to turn. Dr. Shah was a pediatrician who came highly recommended for complex cases from a dear and trusted friend.

Dr. Shah tossed her waist-length brown hair over her shoulder and frowned.

"You've seen a lot of specialists recently, haven't you," she said, her hazel eyes glinting at me, the green flecks in her irises picked up by the green of the exam room walls.

"We believe Sebastian has a very rare neurological visual impairment," I explained calmly, for what seemed like the thousandth time. "We have had a hard time getting a diagnosis."

"Come here," she jerked her head, her smile too wide and

fixed.

I stood up and looked at the graph she'd pulled up for me on her computer. It was a line graph of Sebastian's medical history. The curve of exponential growth was virtually flat for the first fourteen years. The part of the graph Dr. Shah was pointing at so triumphantly was the explosion that happened since January, after we discovered Sebastian's face blindness.

"See?" Dr. Shah posed, Vanna White-like, giving me an unfriendly look.

I gave Sebastian a glance, and he was shrinking into his seat, eyes down. I gathered my dignity and replied calmly.

"Sebastian has been incredibly healthy all his life until this happened," I said, trying not to be defensive. I was quite offended at what Dr. Shah was implying; more so than I could or would explain to this arrogant stranger.

"When we see this," Dr. Shah gestured at the graph. "it's usually *indicative of something.*"

I was quite aware of what that "something" was that Dr. Shah was referring to, but I ignored the unsubtle implication and said, "It is not uncommon when you have a rare condition to have difficulty getting a diagnosis." I tried flattery and smiled. I explained that my friend had recommended her. "She said you were great with complex cases."

Dr. Shah nodded in recognition at the familiar name but was unmoved. She made a big show of asking me to leave the room for Sebastian's examination, as though I would have objected. When I was invited back in five minutes later, Sebastian and I exchanged a look. Dr. Shah looked frustrated and slightly less obnoxious.

"Will you be able to fill Sebastian's prescription for Pristiq?" I asked her.

Her lip curled down and for such a short person, it was remarkable how well she was able to look down her nose at me, seated in the chair that way.

"I don't like to do that," she said pompously, tossing the spectacular curtain of hair again, "but in cases like this, sometimes I have to."

Sebastian and I didn't talk much on our way home. He had his Pristiq prescription filled, and all we could do was wait to go to California and pray.

"Let's go see the baby birds," I suggested. People we knew had a batch of new baby birds.

"Yeah," he said, with genuine enthusiasm. "Let's go."

We went and they showed us the new baby dusky conures. They were such little baby birds, all pin-feathery and helpless. Those lovely wise eyes watched us carefully as we gingerly held each baby bird. They liked to snuggle, and one of them fell asleep in Sebastian's hands.

***

"It's really slow here," Sebastian remarked, shifting around to get comfortable.

My legs were falling asleep from sitting so long. Sebastian and I had embarked on this appointment early. Dr. Drake Anselm's office was located far north of Chicago. Sebastian was silent on the drive. His face was drawn and pale. We arrived about fifteen minutes early for our appointment at three.

Dr. Anselm had a very busy neuro ophthalmology practice. I yawned and tried to ignore the chatty older woman seated next to me as politely as possible. The talkative stranger loved Dr. Anselm, she said. He was the best, she went on. *I don't know if that is going to help us,* I thought, nodding. *Everyone always loves their doctor until the doctor can't diagnose you.* Finally, the woman got called back, and I got a little peace and quiet. It was now almost five o'clock.

I read the news and looked at Facebook. *Everyone has a much more normal life than me,* I thought ruefully. *Comparison is the thief of joy. Don't compare. Many people would trade places with you in a heartbeat,* I thought, and I knew it was true.

At five thirty the office was slowing down. There was one other gentleman sitting in the corner. He looked about seventy, and he was quite sprightly when his name was called. Sebastian and I look at each other and sighed. A few minutes later I heard, "Sebastian!"

Every muscle creaked and both my knees popped when I stood up and stretched. I was trying not to yawn as I walked towards the assistant, Sebastian at my side. The office was empty now as she took us back to the exam room. She asked us a few questions and I told her what we knew, as simply as possible. Trying to condense a ten-hour saga into a five-minute synopsis was not so easy as it may seem. I stuck to the basics.

The young assistant was professional and nonjudgmental. She gave me no indication either way of how she felt about what I was telling her. She took notes on the chart and then smiled.

"Dr. Anselm will be right in with you."

Sebastian and I both took out our phones. I looked around the exam room. It was a very small room, with plain white walls. There were two old framed tacky artworks on the wall in front of me. The seventies-style floral prints hung crookedly in their position on the wall by the door.

Sebastian and I sat in the two brown vinyl visitors' chairs. They were not terribly uncomfortable. There was an optometric chair in the middle, and a small desk with a computer on it to the right. It was quite cramped and the air was stuffy. The whole place smelled like carpet glue, which was weird because the grubby gray swirled carpet was obviously not new. I felt like all the alveoli in my lungs were so sticky, I could taste it. There was no outside ventilation happening in this environmental control system.

I turned my attention back to my phone and checked my email. I had a couple of messages from my baby class mamas. I answered one and was about to answer the one from Jamal's mom when the door came crashing open and an irate, broad-shouldered man with a blond crew cut burst into the tiny exam room. He put his fist in my face and screamed: "Tell me how it's possible he can recognize letters and numbers but not faces! It's all the same channels!"

Fear No Evil

I jerked back in my chair, hands raised protectively, gabbling terrified nonsense, as Dr. Anselm waved his huge fist inches from my nose.

"It's all the same channels!" Dr. Anselm was spitting as he shouted in my face.

Years of training from my home life growing up took over. I sat there and I took it, jabbering helplessly to a strange doctor who had just burst into our exam room screaming without even an introduction.

"Tell me how it's possible!" Dr. Anselm raged. The neuro ophthalmologist's face was red with fury, his lips curled down in rage. His eyes raked over me with hatred and indignation.

I cowered back in my chair, unable to even see Sebastian. I couldn't even look away from this huge and angry man as I stuttered. I don't have any idea what I said. I was frozen to my chair. I felt rather than saw Sebastian next to me, stiff and silent.

Dr. Anselm filled the tiny room with his outrage and his thick, broad shoulders. He was average height but hugely muscular, a body builder obviously. There was no escape. He blocked the door, standing right in front of me. He shouted and raged, confident the office was empty now that it was after six o'clock.

"Tell me how it's possible that he can recognize letters and not faces!" he shouted, again, still waving that meaty fist.

Not getting a satisfactory response from me, he sat himself down on the stool by his computer. He was just four feet away, and he typed with his left hand as he raged with his fisted right.

"It's all the same channels!" he shouted, typing and gesticulating at me at the same time.

"We are here hoping that you can tell us!" I finally managed. "You're the doctor. You tell us how it's possible."

Now, almost two years later, I ask myself why I didn't just leave. The answer was simple. I was raised this way. Running made abuse worse. Be quiet. Be still. Don't contradict. And for goodness' sake, don't cry. So, I didn't. And I didn't call the police, either, because I assumed the police officer would take one look at Sebastian and would never believe he was blind. So, I sat silently while Dr. Anselm gesticulated and raged at me.

Dr. Anselm gave Sebastian a very brief neuro ophthalmology exam, including visual fields, which for Sebastian came out normal. He shouted and waved his clenched fist at me for the entire time we were there. He never stopped waving his right fist at me as he typed and performed the exam. We were there for maybe fifteen minutes, probably less.

There was no one in the office except the one elusive assistant who checked us in. I caught just a glimpse of her as she dodged out the hallway door to the reception area as we moved to the visual fields testing room. She looked scared.

When he finished the visual fields test, Dr. Anselm announced that Sebastian's visual fields were normal, and then sneered that nothing was wrong with Sebastian's vision. I choked out that we were going to the neurology clinic in Southern California on May 15.

"They won't find anything!" he scoffed nastily. "Send me the report!" He laughed sarcastically and walked out of the exam room door.

Sebastian and I barely looked at each other. We didn't speak. As we went through the door back to the reception area, Dr. Anselm banged the door open again and called across the large waiting area.

"I'll see you in six months." He barked a loud, sarcastic laugh and walked out the door.

The elusive assistant was making herself very, very busy behind the front desk. She wouldn't make eye contact with me. I made the appointment.

***

"Hello, you pretty bird, you," Sebastian said.

Kalo the macaw cocked her gorgeous head and looked at

Sebastian with her intelligent eye. She marched her gigantic bird feet in slow motion over the top of the finch cage. She was a primary-colored Godzilla. Finches fluttered excitedly while her long blue tail passed overhead like a very slow-moving jet plane. The little birds clearly expect radioactive flames at any moment.

The large, intelligent bird reached with her ferocious beak to grasp the mesquite tree perch next to the cage. She pulled herself up with her beak, her large taloned feet slowly reaching and grasping at the branches. She seized a wooden toy hanging from the rope fishing net strung across the rear wall. She held it with one scaly claw and crunched down. Wood shards rained down on the sand below the bird perch. She considered Sebastian as she crunched.

"Cookie," the bird suggested. She looked to see if a treat was coming. It was not, so she took another crunch out of the wooden toy.

"You are such a pretty bird," Sebastian said again as he took another photo.

The two green baby dusky conures were much more active today. It was shocking how a week or two could make a difference. We each got one baby bird to hold. The little pin feathers on the head made mine look comical. The little feathers poked straight up out of the skin of its head, like they were surprised to be there. The little baby birds, just a little bigger than parakeets, were very cuddly and affectionate.

Sebastian and I took turns passing each little bird back and forth. One of them obviously preferred our company. I bought it for Sebastian. I would do anything to end the constant sadness and depression. The baby bird was so all-consuming in its adoration of Sebastian, and the feeling was mutual. It was too little to come home, so we left it there to be hand-fed until it fledged and was completely weaned onto solid food.

I hadn't been able to find any words to comfort Sebastian as we left Dr. Anselm's office. After the shocking shouting session, Sebastian and I sat silently in the car. I had no words. He had no words.

Finally, I said, "Let's get donuts."

As we waited in the drive-thru, I tried to find something to say. I looked at him, sitting beside me, hopeless with despair and humiliation.

"I am sorry for the way that man acted. He had no right to treat either one of us that way, and I'm sorry you had to see that. That should never have happened." I paused, looking for any reaction from Sebastian. He looked at his hands. I continued. "That man is afraid. He is to be pitied, not feared. He had four months to prepare for our appointment, and in that time, he made the choice to refuse to look, or learn, or read. I told the receptionist you had prosopagnosia and environmental agnosia when I made the appointment."

Sebastian's eyes flashed. He clenched his fists and with his jaw tight, he answered: "Yeah, if he had even Googled face blindness, he would have found Oliver Sacks and Chuck Close. He would know that it's not 'all the same channels.'"

His voice dripped with sarcasm. The bitterness in Sebastian's voice made my eyes sting. I swallowed hard and willed the tears back.

"Exactly. Instead, he made a choice out of fear. He is so fearful of what he doesn't know that he spent four months planning to verbally abuse and threaten a woman in front of her own child. That is not okay, and when I am finished getting a diagnosis for you, I will take action."

"You don't have to, Mom."

"I will; I just need to take care of you first." I quoted Psalm 23.

"Mom, I don't believe in this stuff. I am not a Christian."

"I know, sweetie. You don't have to believe just because I do. I think it helps me to understand things."

Sebastian looked straight ahead. "I just don't like the idea of life after death."

"Really? Why?"

"I'm not sure," he looked at his hands again. "I guess I just feel tired."

I inhaled and looked at him from the side of my eye.

"You always said that I'm an old soul," he continued. "I'm just done. When I die, I don't want to come back."

"Like reincarnation?" I asked.

"Yeah, I sometimes feel like I've done this before."

"Maybe you have. Maybe you'll come back as a bird next time." That got a smile.

"It would be an improvement."

"I used to dream of flying, before all my dreams turned to houses."

"That would be nice."

"What are you going to name your baby bird?"

"Mimi?"

"Love it."

Mimi loved her name too. We went to visit her every day we were able to, which was about four days per week. Sebastian was getting way more confident navigating around Chicago with help, thanks to the marvelous Kaitlyn Peters. We practiced his routes around the art school campus, and he was getting better at finding his way around, but he couldn't navigate by himself yet.

I regularly saw him walk into traffic still. It almost always happened when somebody jaywalked. Sebastian saw the motion of the jaywalker and followed automatically, not realizing the person he followed had scooted through a gap in traffic; a car was coming right at him, and he couldn't see it. I yanked him from the jaws of death on a regular basis. I cursed our quiet neighborhood and very sleepy street.

One extremely hot day in May, as we practiced walking Sebastian's routes between the different campus buildings and dorms, Sebastian went completely blind. Seeing him become unable to read his phone to navigate was terrifying. Sebastian and I had walked about three miles that day in ninety-five-degree weather. We had made a point to bring our water bottles and we both were well hydrated.

Sebastian correctly entered the address for the occupational therapy center into Google Maps on his phone, and he led the way to the bus stop by following the directions on his phone. The heat and humidity were overpowering. As we walked, suddenly Sebastian became agitated.

"I can't read my phone, Mom." His face was panicky. "I can't see what it says."

Fortunately, we had made it to the stop just as the bus pulled up. We asked the bus driver if it was the correct route, and it was. On the twenty-minute air-conditioned bus ride, Sebastian's vision recovered slightly as he cooled off.

I had another memory then of Sebastian at age two playing in the front yard on a very hot day. I remember him being very fussy and crying. I remembered thinking he didn't seem to be able to regulate his body temperature very well. From that time on, we avoided playing outside in the extreme heat unless there was water involved. We had sprinklers, a hot tub out back on Moby Deck, and a huge inflatable water slide he loved to play on.

Now I knew that being overheated affected Sebastian's vision, but I did not know how. The terror of thinking of him, completely blind, alone in the city, was overwhelming for both of us. I knew that the excellent occupational therapy for navigation Sebastian had been receiving from Kaitlyn Peters was not enough. Sebastian needed white-cane training in case he went completely blind again and I wasn't with him.

***

I sat in the empty waiting room impatiently waiting for Sebastian's last vision therapy session with Dr. Alabaster to be over. After ten weeks of vision therapy, I was hoping we'd finally get an actual diagnosis and some guidance on what steps we needed to take to get Sebastian the orientation and mobility training he so desperately needed. Surely this doctor had guided other families through the process of getting white-cane training. I felt my hope rise.

Finally, Sebastian and Dr. Alabaster came out from the back

room and we sat together in the comfortable and empty waiting area. Dr. Alabaster lounged casually, legs crossed comfortably in the chair next to Sebastian. Her mahogany eyes crinkled as she smiled. She had a chart showing that Sebastian's eye muscle strength had improved, so I would know that all the eye crossing and uncrossing had achieved something, but there was no change to his acuity or Sebastian's ability to recognize things.

"So," I asked politely. "Do we have a diagnosis?"

Dr. Alabaster put her arm around Sebastian, and with motherly concern and as kindly as possible said, "Sebastian is noncompliant." I blinked, stunned, and Dr. Alabaster said, "He could see if only he would try harder."

Sebastian was rightfully and obviously offended, but he kept his opinions to himself and listened respectfully to the doctor. I was proud of his self-restraint. I knew from my years of teaching middle school that many teens would have been much, much less polite than my son was. I collected myself, and I very politely reminded this doctor of our very first visit.

"Sebastian is probably one of the most cooperative and compliant teens you could ever meet," I reminded Dr. Alabaster politely. "He has never had a detention, or been in trouble at home, or at a friend's house, or in the community."

How does she not know this fact? I wondered. *We went over all of this at our first appointment.* It was clear Dr. Alabaster didn't remember, or perhaps never listened in the first place. She blinked those liquid mahogany eyes and looked vaguely surprised.

"We know he's unusually cooperative because of his fear of getting lost from the environmental agnosia," I continued. "He stuck close to us, and his friends, because his life depended on it," I said, gaining a little steam. "In fact, all of that information about Sebastian's good character is documented in the neuro psych evaluation I gave you on our first appointment."

Dr. Alabaster looked surprised and guilty. I asked her how Sebastian was supposed to see if he was having difficulty.

"He just needs to focus and use other channels."

"Can you tell me what these other channels might be?" I asked, genuinely curious what her response might be.

I'd been telling Dr. Alabaster about Sebastian's verbal visual processing for ten weeks. I was deeply interested in her response. She could not give me any explanation of what these other channels could have been, but Dr. Alabaster assured me confidently that "there are other channels." She obviously had no idea what they were.

I have to give Dr. Alabaster credit because at least she was nice. She was trying, and she genuinely didn't know the answers. She was neither unkind nor abusive, she just didn't know. Despite that niceness, it was still devastating to Sebastian to be mischaracterized so badly. Every week, he did his very best, as he did his best at everything. He was a perfectionist, and to be called noncompliant, like a juvenile delinquent, really hurt him.

We parted ways courteously. I asked Dr. Alabaster to send the final report to the neurology clinic in California. California was our only hope. Sebastian was extremely bitter, and I couldn't blame him. I was bitter too, and I was frustrated.

Every single night I sat with him and we talked.

"I will not stop. I will not leave you. I will not quit. I will never, ever quit until we get this figured out. The clinic in California will help us."

"I hope so." There was no hope on his face.

"There is no better place to go," I said, willing him to believe. "People from all over the world go to the neurology clinic there. If anyone can help us, it will be them. They know we are coming all the way from Illinois. They would not bring us out there if they weren't going to help us."

California

"We're really here," Sebastian said.

He looked around the shabby hotel lobby. It was May 13, 2017, and Eric, Sebastian, and I were finally in California. The hotel was an independent place that dated from the seventies and was bizarrely decorated around a corn theme. Corn artwork, corn posters, and fake corn in dusty artificial wreaths lined the hallways and the elevator vestibule. We had a late dinner and then went to bed.

"I am so glad to be here," I said to Eric as we were lying in the dark room. "It feels like we've been waiting for this forever."

Eric put his arm around me as we lay quietly in the dark. I had talked with both Lukas and Gala Brooks before we left. Neither of them had been able to find a local orientation and mobility specialist willing to give Sebastian white-cane training. This was our last chance to get Sebastian help.

This is one of the best neurology departments in the world, I thought, feeling the scratchy sheets against my neck. I brought Big Squishy and the Lunk, but I was using the too-soft hotel pillow for my arthritic knees. I wished I'd brought the Knee Pillow, as my right knee knocked the other painfully through the thin stuffing. There wasn't room in the luggage.

I went through my mental checklist. I had shared everything we knew about Sebastian's verbal visual processing in writing with the clinic; each discovery as we made it. My case was clearly and exactly articulated. I had left nothing to chance.

We had finally made it. I felt my hope rise as I lay there in the quiet hotel room. We would finally have a diagnosis for the school. Orientation and mobility training would come next. Sebastian would start white-cane training; if he got overheated again, he would have some safety skills for when his vision was at its worst. Even better, drivers would see his white cane and have a visible signal that he could not see them when he was crossing the street.

"Tomorrow! Tomorrow!" My unhelpful soundtrack teased

me. I hate that song. I could not fall asleep.

The alarm clock startled me awake. We got ready and went downstairs to try the free continental breakfast. Everyone was jittery with a weird excitement.

"It feels like Christmas morning," Sebastian observed cheerfully over his oatmeal. "Like, Christmas in some alternate universe where going to the doctor is really great."

He was simultaneously sarcastic about the doctors and genuinely hopeful about the day. I nodded in complete agreement. My heart surged at his cautious optimism. *We've got this,* I thought to myself.

Out loud, I said "It's going to be okay. We are in the right place. It just took us a while to find it."

We tidied up the remains of our breakfast, all of us bristling with excitement and nerves, and headed towards the elevator to get our coats before heading out to the appointment. As we were waiting in the cramped elevator vestibule, Eric gestured vaguely towards the pool doors on our left.

"Look! It's a croton," I heard him say. The plant by the pool door was a spikey snake plant like the one on our mantelpiece at home. Puzzled, I corrected him. "That's a snake plant."

Eric stood with his back to me in the tiny elevator lobby. "It's a corn cob," Eric said, speaking more clearly now and waving again towards the pool doors.

I was completely bewildered and annoyed.

"That is not a corn cob," I said emphatically, now completely confused. "It's a snake plant."

Eric turned, his face cross. "That is not a snake plant."

"Yes, it is. It's just like the one on our mantelpiece."

"It is not a snake plant." Eric's voice was clipped and tight. He hated travel, and the stress made him crabby.

"What are you talking about? It is a snake plant. I bought it, I know what it is." My voice rose in irritation, my mood matching Eric's now.

Sebastian was looking at me like I was an alien, his lips twisted into a frown.

"What?" I asked, my annoyance rising even more.

Eric stepped to the side and very clearly pointed to the poster by the elevator. It was a wrinkled and dog-eared picture of a corn cob with the words "Welcome to California" printed in large blue letters across the top.

"That's a corn cob."

That's all it took. I was crying/laughing.

"I thought you said 'croton!'"

Sebastian stared at me, and then he burst out laughing too. Eric's face darkened, and he scowled.

"I said 'It's a corn cob,'" he said, more than a little defensively, which made me laugh harder.

"I know!" I said, gasping for breath. "But you were waving your hand towards that!" I pointed at the plastic plant sitting sadly by the glass pool door. The elevator door opened and two bewildered senior citizens, a husband and wife, stepped cautiously past us. The woman gave me the eyebrow raise as we slid past them. Sebastian and I laughed hysterically, and every time we made eye contact, we got louder and more obnoxious.

Sebastian was laughing at what an idiot I was, and I was laughing at myself. Eric finally gave in and grinned, and then led the way back down the hallway shaking his head; Sebastian's and my uncouth noise in a hotel hallway was too much to bear for my polite husband.

Months of fear and frustration came pouring out in helpless gales as we followed him down the hallway, careless of the other travelers. Sebastian and I were so loopy and relieved to be there that our sporadic laughing fits continued in the car on the short ride over to the clinic. Even Eric finally joined in from the sheer ridiculousness of our hilarity.

"Oh, my God," I laughed breathlessly again, for the fourth time. I was slap happy. "We've become Abbott and Costello!"

"Who are Abbott and Costello?" Sebastian asked, his face flushed from all the hilarity.

It was rare that I knew something he didn't. It was the one benefit of being older than him. I loved it when I could whip something out and surprise him. I was slightly triumphant in my temporary advantage over him.

"Who's on first, What's on second, I Don't Know's on third," Eric interjected. I smiled at him and he smiled back.

"What?" Sebastian asked, confused. He didn't know the quote. I had been deficient in teaching him the classics, I could see.

"That's exactly what I said," Eric continued, answering Sebastian's question. "Who's on first, *What's* on second, I Don't Know's on third."

"Google 'Who's on First,'" I said.

Sebastian finished watching the old comedy skit just as we pulled into the parking lot. We were all smiling as we walked into the neurology clinic and were welcomed back right away. We were sitting there in this big but very ordinary exam room for about five minutes, waiting, anxious and excited. Our journey was over. We were going to get a diagnosis and move on with our lives. When we got home, I could call the school and schedule our meeting with the team. My thoughts were spinning.

Sebastian was sitting quietly, looking thoughtful and optimistic. We made eye contact, and he drawled laconically, "That's not a corncob, it's a snake plant."

That's all it took. Hysterical laughter came pealing out from both of us. Eric looked on amused while Sebastian rolled in his chair. I grabbed a tissue from the desk beside me, and I had just passed one to Sebastian when the exam room door opened and a tiny, wrinkled man with a thick, full gray walrus mustache peeked in at the commotion. *It's the Lorax,* I thought. *We are saved!*

"Hello," Dr. Adam J. Rentschler said.

I hurriedly blotted my traitor eyes and caught my breath, still giggling madly. I caught a glimpse of Dr. Rentschler as he strode past us, his eyes flashing with amusement over each of our faces. He turned and stood by the computer at the end of the room. His tonsured gray hair rimmed his shiny skull, and his impressive steely mustache bristled as he grinned. A flash of amusement sparked his kind eyes, a micro expression.

It was his voice that did me in. Dr. Rentschler was one of those very small men who surprise you with their deep basso profundo voices. *He's a Russian bass,* I thought, surprised. *Where does all that sound come from?* His voice was so resonant and clear that I could tell he was a singer. My hope surged.

Just from that one single hello, my mind was racing with optimism. *He was a musician! He would know the neuroscience of music and the brain. He would understand how Sebastian had all normal developmental milestones even though he was almost completely blind.*

He will have read my long explanations of how Sebastian had intensive music therapy by accident of having a music teacher for a mother. He would know that children who have music and movement in early childhood have better balance and proprioception than those who don't. He knows these children have better gross and fine motor skills and, on average, a 20 percent increase in IQ. He knows!

My zygomatic lift is activated, I thought bizarrely as I smiled through my tears. I was about to say hello when I finally heard his words. Dr. Rentschler was addressing all of us. He stood by his computer desk, his spine drawn up to maximize his very minimal height. All traces of humor was extinguished from those kindly eyes. His face was a mask of deep pity and concern.

"It's a good thing you can laugh at times like this."

Sebastian went white and I collapsed against the back of my chair.

Dr. Rentschler proceeded to pull up his homemade prosopagnosia test to check Sebastian's ability to recognize faces. He asked Sebastian to stand beside him, and then one by one, he showed Sebastian photos of famous people. There was Beyoncé, Oprah, Taylor Swift, and other celebrities, including President Obama. Sebastian got seven out of ten correct.

Calmly and very, very kindly, Dr. Rentschler explained that Sebastian "can't have prosopagnosia with a score of seven out of ten." He said, "People with prosopagnosia can't recognize faces at all."

"Sebastian isn't recognizing faces here," I politely corrected him. "He uses verbal characteristics to identity everything and everyone." Clearly, Dr. Rentschler must have read my notes, and he just didn't want to believe them. He was obviously not impressed. I pressed on anyway.

"Sebastian recognizes me with tall/blonde/glasses," I explained, politely. "He has verbal characteristics for everything; that includes objects, familiar people, *and* celebrities. If he wasn't able to recognize people with these verbal descriptors, we would have noticed a long time ago that there was something wrong."

Dr. Rentschler calmly explained to us again that "it's just not possible for a person with prosopagnosia to recognize faces."

"He isn't recognizing the faces," I repeated, hoping to drill understanding into this concrete block of obstinance with repetition. I spoke with passion, but politely. "What's actually telling is that he missed Taylor Swift. His best friend April was a Taylor Swift fan growing up. Sebastian has seen Taylor Swift's face millions of times on his friend's concert T-shirts, posters, and buttons. If he had a typical ability to recognize faces, he would have recognized Taylor Swift right away. He guessed Marilyn Monroe. They're both often shown with blonde hair and red lipstick. He can't tell the two of them apart."

"I can't recognize any faces," Sebastian said honestly. "I can't recognize mine. I assumed that everyone was like this. I didn't know I was different."

I felt my face flush with pride in my son for speaking up for himself. I watched in wonder as Sebastian, who had been insulted, screamed at, and threatened by small, ignorant, frightened doctors, stood up for himself. With great dignity and articulation, a teenager who had been denigrated by doctors so fearful of nonconformity and the very idea or possibility of vision without recognition that they chose to terrorize their own patient: a child.

Sebastian stood and spoke the truth. He was tall and calm; his voice was confident and without arrogance. He fought to be seen by a man who refused to listen, or learn, or read; a doctor without imagination whose curiosity and sense of wonder died back in medical school; a man who refused to see what was right before his eyes. My son patiently and completely explained in extraordinary and exhaustive detail his own visual processing. Sebastian was convincing and heartfelt.

The artist Frederick Franck's extraordinary words from his book *The Zen of Seeing: Seeing/Drawing as Meditation* came to me as I watched my fifteen-year-old stand before this oblivious man with dignity and extraordinary composure. Sebastian tried to make himself visible. He tried with all his will to be seen.

> *"Millions of people, unseeing, joyless, blunder through life in their half-sleep, hitting, kicking, and killing what they have barely perceived. They have never learned to SEE, or they have forgotten that man has eyes to SEE, to experience.*
>
> *When a man no longer experiences, the organs of his inner life wither away. Alone or in herds, he goes on binges of violence and destruction.*
>
> *Looking and seeing both start with sense perception, but there the similarity ends."* - Frederick Franck

Dr. Rentschler looked at Sebastian standing before him, but he refused to see him. *Whose brain machine is broken?* I asked myself silently. *Who is the one who lacks perception?*

Sebastian stood, a child of fifteen, and said, "I couldn't recognize any of the faces. I guessed it was Obama because it was an African-American man, dressed in a navy suit, with an American flag behind him and a flag lapel pin." He paused briefly and thought. "It was the wide smile that clinched it."

Dr. Rentschler looked at Sebastian and for a moment, I saw a flash of belief; a fraction of a second of belief in his eyes. Then he blinked and chose not to see him.

"He's using context and salient characteristics," I explained, willing this man to understand.

"It's just not possible for people with prosopagnosia to

recognize faces," the doctor said with finality.

Case closed. Eyes closed.

But the case wasn't closed yet, oh no. There were other doctors at the clinic for us to see, who would all look at us but not see us. It was immediately apparent that they had come to a communal decision before we arrived that the diagnosis was "Mom is crazy, and she's afraid to put her kid in driver's ed-itis."

We were in California for three days. Dr. Rentschler offered us an MRI to pacify the lunatics. Sebastian had had a couple of brain scans since the concussion, all normal. We had sent the imaging along before we arrived, so he knew it. Dr. Rentschler said there was something called a SPECT scan, but: "We only use it on elderly dementia patients, so there are no fifteen-year-old brains in the library of past patients to compare" Sebastian to. For that reason, he said, "There would be no way to tell if Sebastian's brain is normal or not."

"The SPECT scan is useless. It's a nuclear medicine test," Dr. Rentschler said, making it sound very dangerous, "so you should really spare him."

With all of Sebastian's drug reactions, I struggled, and then said no to the SPECT scan. Because I had never received the full panel of genetic testing results, I had no idea what Sebastian might react to, and nobody at the clinic was helpful.

"We're so, so sorry." Dr. Rentschler dripped compassion on the second day. "Someone in the office messed up your MRI appointment. Can you come back next week?"

I was so traumatized that it was more than a year later when I realized no one messed up our MRI schedule, they were just trying to encourage us to go home. I was so desperate for help, we made the trip home, rearranged our pet sitters, and then we came back to California the following week.

I was holding on by a thread, hoping against hope that the stronger MRI would reveal a lesion that had gone undetected, and that perhaps surgery could fix Sebastian's vision. While we waited, we met with a neuropsychologist, who did another battery of visual-spatial testing on Sebastian. The neuropsychologist told us Sebastian had average visual-spatial scores, so he had average vision. The end. There could be no allowance for the genius verbal abilities to be skewing the visual spatial scores. I disagreed logically, calmly.

"Sebastian is able to describe his own visual processing. We are lucky he has the intellectual ability to do so," I explained. "His visual memory is not average, it's almost nonexistent."

"That's not possible," the neuropsychologist said, arrogantly. This doctor had numbers on a paper, and that was all this person needed.

"How do you explain Sebastian's extraordinary math performance on all standardized tests with such low visual-spatial scores? He's never been tutored or coached. Shouldn't he have difficulty with math with scores like that?"

The neuropsychologist shrugged and sat silently.

"He cried every day for three months before he went to middle school," I argued. "He told us he was afraid he would get lost, every single night. Why would he do that if there wasn't a real fear?"

The neuropsychologist looked me in the eye, and with a slow, sly significance said, "I don't know..." and then looked me up and down, mouth tight. I saw it, and to my immense agony, so did Sebastian.

My mouth dropped open in horror. In front of my child, this arrogant monster had made such an insinuation. I tried again. I refused to stop trying.

"Sebastian can't recognize his environment, we know that," I continued, desperately. "He needs a diagnosis so he can get orientation and mobility services through his school. We have seen him go completely blind when he is overheated. We walked three miles in the heat, and he couldn't even read his phone. Thank God I was with him at the time. He depends on Google Maps to navigate. If he can't even read his phone his life is in danger. He could have been hit by the bus if I hadn't been with him."

The neuropsychologist looked at me like I was a lunatic and

said, very primly, “You should put him on a bike in heavy traffic. That will help him to get used to all the traffic.”

“I can’t put him on a bike in heavy traffic.” I gasped out loud, thinking *We have dodged so many bullets already*. “He could be killed! We almost put him in driver’s ed. The only reason we didn’t was because of the concussion. He would be dead now if we hadn’t figured out what was wrong.”

“It’s perfectly safe to enroll him in driver’s ed,” the doctor said, like I was four and I needed a lollipop.

“It is not safe to put him in driver’s ed. He has almost no visual memory. Look, we aren’t asking for medication or surgery. We are asking for a couple of weeks of orientation and mobility so Sebastian can work with a white cane, in the certain event he loses all vision again while traveling independently. It’s a minor request.”

“No. He has average vision. He doesn’t need it.”

“Please, he needs to see a neuro ophthalmologist!” I was shamelessly begging at this point. “I know he has a neurological visual impairment.”

“No.”

“Please, I’m begging you to help us.”

“No!” the doctor shouted in my face and then stood and without another word, we were dismissed.

On our final day in California we met again with Dr. Rentschler. He was smarmy and condescending. He brought up the images of Sebastian’s brain from the MRI. He said they took tons of pictures, and he extolled how beautiful and perfect Sebastian’s brain was as he scrolled through the imaging.

“Everything is normal,” he said reassuringly to the psychotic patients. “There is no possible way he can have a neurological visual impairment and a normal brain scan.” He looked kindly at all of us and said. “It is perfectly safe for Sebastian to take driver’s ed.”

“No,” I disagreed firmly. “I will not allow that unless he can pass the evaluation for drivers with visual impairment at our local hospital. There’s a program for visually impaired drivers near us. I won't let him drive unless he can pass their safety screening."

Dr. Rentschler sighed and gave in, just to get rid of us. He was tired of the crazy lady and wanted to go get lunch. In his deep basso profundo voice he said to us nicely that we "need family therapy" and that he truly believed "Sebastian's vision will improve with therapy and medication." He said he "has seen it happen that anti-anxiety medication cures vision problems."

I knew this was bullshit, so I asked him, miraculously without any sarcasm, "Will it also cure his diagnosed, documented auditory processing disorder?" I asked it nicely. We were all so polite.

"No," he said. "Curing the vision is like a side effect of the medication."

Exhausted and defeated, I asked, "Do you really think that?" I wanted an honest answer.

"Yes."

On the way home I texted Lukas. "They said it's psychogenic."

Lukas replied, outraged: How do they explain this? How do they explain that?

"They didn't," I typed back. "They didn't answer any of our questions. They just treated us like escapees from the asylum."

Sightless Flight

Coming home was devastating; I will not write about it. The day after we arrived home, I found a low-vision clinic in Boston. It was at someplace called the Perkins School for the Blind. I called the number, and I started off okay.

"My son has a neurological visual impairment and a normal MRI. Has anyone ever *heard* of this?!?" I was sobbing by the end of the sentence.

The nice person on the phone took my number and said he'd have someone call me back. *It's finally happened,* I thought. *I truly have gone insane. I will never hear from anyone.* A day or two later I was doing laundry and tidying up the kitchen when my phone rang. It was Lukas.

"Hello," I said, shakily.

Lukas's calm and reassuring baritone voice barely reached me. He said he had reached out to Jim Deremeik, the head of rehabilitation at the Johns Hopkins Eye Clinic.

"Jim's a busy man. He wants to talk to you right now."

"Thank you, Lukas. I'll call him right away." I tried to pull myself together.

"Don't cry when you talk to him."

Jim Deremeik's deep baritone voice was friendly, very professional, and inquisitive. He asked important questions about Sebastian and his ability to navigate. Lukas had clearly prepared him.

"I just don't want my kid to get hit by a bus," I said, feeling my face flush. "He has a fabulous OT, but he still walks into traffic. He needs O&M. I have seen Sebastian go completely blind when he's overheated. He's got to have some white-cane training in the event it happens again when I am not with him. He needs to be able to travel independently."

Jim did an extraordinary thing then. He offered to enroll me in a class on something called "Cortical Visual Impairment." I wondered at the new term and felt my own incredulity that Sebastian's condition had a name. Cortical visual impairment!

I had been correctly using the term prosopagnosia to describe the symptom of face blindness for five months now at dozens of doctor appointments and had never once even heard the name of my son's condition. I was stunned and shocked that in all my research I had never found the term cortical, or cerebral impairment either.

It must be something about the way the search engine worked, I decided. There was so little information online about Sebastian's condition. As I processed this new discovery and wondered at how the Google search engine worked, Jim explained that the course was usually $150, but he was donating it to me free of charge. Jim explained that the class would help me to "be a better advocate for my son."

I didn't entirely manage not to cry.

***

On Saturday morning, I began the class on CVI, entitled *Understanding Cortical Visual Impairment in Children,* at Emerald Events. It was Memorial Day weekend, 2017. The course was taught by Dr. Gordon Dutton, a pediatric ophthalmologist and professor emeritus of visual sciences at Glasgow Caledonian University in Scotland. Dr. Dutton's Scottish accent and genial eyes captivated my attention. He said CVI had been identified as the number-one cause of visual impairment in children in the developed world over ten years ago, and still didn't have a diagnostic code.

Mouth open in shock, I sat at the kitchen table and stared. I clicked the screen to restart the lecture and listened again. Cerebral/cortical visual impairment was not rare, but common. In fact, I learned CVI was more common than ocular blindness. There were tens of thousands of people here in the United States who had CVI.

I sat back, stunned by my outrage. Everything I had read and been told about Sebastian's condition being extremely rare was wrong.

I searched for CVI Facebook groups, and there they were, hidden in plain sight. Thousands of families, just like us, desperately searching for a doctor with knowledge. Mothers and fathers, searching for help with accommodations at school and at home; trying desperately to understand their child's condition. Terrible cries for help, when every doctor they saw knew nothing about CVI, or worse—and more frequently—confidently gave them false information.

The frustration and sadness for all these families is all so unnecessary, I thought, as I sat there holding my phone and scrolling through one agonized post after another. Our search for help was no longer about just my son, my child. Something had to change. I dove into Dr. Dutton's course on CVI.

I learned the visual system and I saw how light traveled through the lens of the eye to the retina, where it is passed through the transparent lining of axons, to the ganglion cells, to the bipolar cells, and on to the rods and cones. I could picture the rods and cones receiving images and shifting them to an electrical signal. This signal passed through the optic nerves through the optic chiasm to the lateral geniculate nuclei (LGN), which functioned as the relay stations of the visual system. From the LGN, the electrical signals were sent to the occipital lobes in the back of the brain where the signals were processed.

I learned about the function of the occipital lobes in the back of the brain, and then there it was: The temporal lobes of the brain are where images are stored, making memories for comparison.

Dr. Dutton clearly laid out where in the brain each type of recognition occurred: faces, places, objects, biological forms, words, letters, numbers, and shapes. Each were processed in a distinct and already identified area. Years of research had all been completed, all understandable, all mapped out. I devoured the information.

Professor Dutton explained everything in detail about the dorsal and ventral streams of the brain. At first, I had to think of the dorsal fin of a shark to keep the two parts of the brain straight. Sebastian had both dorsal- and ventral-stream impairment.

I had it. No, Dr. Anslem, they are not "ALL THE SAME CHANNELS!" Not by far. I shook my fist at him mentally.

On and on, I couldn't learn enough. None of this information was difficult to understand or complicated. It was presented in as straightforward, articulate, and logical a manner as was possible. Hysterical laughter bubbled out of me as I read. A music teacher could understand this and learn it all in one weekend. The absurdity of the lot of it made me want to laugh and cry at the same time.

Why wasn't this information being taught to the doctors?

I studied the upper midbrain, where reflex vision happens; the reflex that makes a person blink in time to keep things from hitting the eye before it's even consciously seen. I also learned about the posterior parietal lobes that map the visual scene to plan our movement, to search, and to give attention. I thought about Sebastian's typical developmental milestones and wondered. I knew we had a photo of Sebastian reaching to grab Eric's tongue when he was a baby.

I was positive Sebastian was born with CVI, and that my preeclampsia and subsequent brush with death at his birth was the cause. After the nurse bolused my epidural, I had coded. My blood pressure had dropped to 40/26, and I received a six-inch needle of epinephrine to my heart while I was unconscious. That injection saved my life, but now I suspected that I'd had a mild stroke. After all, Sebastian had a partial photographic memory for text that he inherited from me. Mine disappeared when he was born, and I didn't miss it for several years because I wasn't writing research papers. Busy raising a child and trying to scrub bathtub crayon out of grout (which is not easy, Crayola!), I didn't connect the two events.

My mom friends and I commiserated about our new ditzy mom brains at play group; I thought everyone felt the same vagueness I did. I had joked for years that Sebastian had sucked my photographic memory right out of me. I had blamed it on age and distraction. Now I thought that we had both suffered a stroke from lack of oxygen. In my imagination, I heard the blare of the code-blue alarm as I sat there at the kitchen table, and I saw the anesthesiologist's face, assuring me: "It's okay, close your eyes."

They told us Sebastian got a nine on his Apgar score.

I can still hear Eric saying, "That's an A!"

There's no way Sebastian truly got a nine on his Apgar, I thought as I sat there in front of the computer watching Professor Dutton speak, eloquently brilliant. I remembered taking Sebastian back to the doctor for each of his postnatal appointments. At each one, I expressed my concerns about how much Sebastian was sleeping, and at each one, my concerns were pooh-poohed.

"You just have a very sleepy baby," they said.

Thank goodness I'm a music teacher. I shuddered to think what the quality of Sebastian's life would have looked like without music and movement therapy as an intervention. I snapped back to attention and continued watching Dr. Gordon Dutton's fascinating lecture on CVI, and there was the answer to my most frustrating question: How could Sebastian have CVI and a normal MRI? Dr. Gordon Dutton explained succinctly that many people with CVI have a normal-appearing brain scan.

"Taking a history is often more effective than an MRI scan" for diagnosing CVI, Dr. Dutton said. In fact, 10 percent of cerebral palsy patients also have a normal-appearing brain scan, and the percentages for patients with CVI are believed to be about the same, he explained. Pathologies were often missed, particularly in the superior posterior parietal area on both sides of the brain.

I hooted with triumph. "Ah hah! There it is! Eric, check this out!"

Eric came over to see what I was thrilling over.

"You can have a normal-appearing brain scan and CVI," I told him. "An MRI only measures the structure of the brain; it can't show the function. Sebastian's brain injury was years ago, and so it doesn't show."

I hugged Eric, and we swayed there for a moment in the

kitchen.

"You were right," Eric said.

"Thank you," I said. "I know."

I kept going. I learned about strabismus and amblyopia. Sebastian had a slight exotropic strabismus that could result in amblyopia and permanent vision loss, as the brain would stop paying attention to the signals from the lazy eye if not treated. *Why did nobody tell us?* I fumed. Lazy eye! Seriously.

I mean, I get it. Sebastian's chameleon gaze was subtle, but it wasn't invisible, and how many times had I pointed it out? I heard my mother's voice in the back of my head: "I don't know what's wrong with everyone. Everyone else is crazy."

I laughed and cried at the table.

I learned about blindsight. There were other people in addition to Sebastian walking around blind, not bumping into things. Then I remembered. Blindsight. The word triggered a memory I had completely forgotten. One of my coworkers at my first teaching job in Lombard had had a child with blindsight twenty years ago, and the word brought my memory of this extraordinary person back to me.

A lovely young woman, this teen was diagnosed with autism and blindsight. She was a savant and could count things like cards. She walked through my classroom as easily as an otter in a kelp bed. She moved about so easily that I had forgotten she was blind until hearing the word twenty years later.

I finished the coursework excitedly. There were two types of blindsight, low level and high. The high-level dorsal stream vision was unconscious but ***could be rendered conscious.*** The vision could be fatigable and intermittent. It can vary from day to day and moment to moment. Triumphant, I sat up straight.

"This is why Sebastian went completely blind that day in the heat! Visual tiring is real!"

Eric laughed. "Finding all the facts, aren't you?"

"Yes. It's all here, everything."

I waited impatiently for the Memorial Day weekend to be over. I sent Jim Deremeik a thank-you email for the course. I got an A.

"What should I do next?" I asked, after listing all the things that I knew were wrong with my son's vision, using all the correct terminology. It was a long list.

An email response arrived, with two local doctors listed, and the note that they "might be able to help us." The doctors' phone numbers and emails were provided.

After some Googling I chose the doctor who was associated with a major hospital. I knew there was not a cure for Sebastian's vision, but I was hopeful there might be some sort of therapy. I knew now from taking Professor Dutton's course on CVI that Sebastian could develop amblyopia from strabismus and that he could lose what little vision he had if I couldn't find a doctor to treat it. Sebastian needed treatment to save what little vision he had.

I called the first doctor.

"Good morning! Dr. Wister's office. How may I help you?"

"Hi, my name is Stephanie Duesing and we have only recently discovered that my son has CVI. He is fifteen, and it's a very late discovery. I was told by Jim Deremeik, the head of rehabilitation at the Johns Hopkins Eye Clinic, to call you."

The receptionist was cheerful. "We can see you today."

I could not believe my ears. Today, and after all we'd been through. I inhaled sharply and laughed out loud. Jubilation and relief flooded through me. Finally, after all these months, we were coming to the end of this medical nightmare.

"Are you kidding me?" I asked, nervous but hopeful. "That's incredible. Thank you."

"It's like you have the secret passcode," the receptionist agreed, amused.

"What time?" I held my breath while I waited for her response.

"Three thirty," she said nicely. "It's our only opening."

We had OT that afternoon. I deflated. "We have occupational therapy today at three and we need to cancel twenty-four hours in advance," I said. "I'm so sorry. I would really like to come in today. We've had a hard time getting a diagnosis, and Dr. Wister comes highly recommended."

"I completely understand," the receptionist said sweetly. "The next available is in two weeks."

"We'll take it."

I immediately sat down and emailed this new doctor, telling her exactly what Sebastian's symptoms were using all the correct terminology, and, with permission from the people involved, I explained who had recommended we see her.

***

"Are you ready?" Sebastian asked, nipping at my heels. "I've got everything loaded in the car."

"Did you pack your art supplies?" I teased. It was Father's Day, and we were headed out to drop Sebastian at the School of the Art Institute for his two-week Early College Program oil painting class.

"Yes." He smiled. His handsome face was suffused with anticipation. We had enjoyed this past week making art supply purchases at Dick Blick. He grinned. "I've got my painting case and all my stuff."

I wiped off the counter.

"Come on, let's go," Eric said, grabbing Sebastian's suitcase and heading out the door.

The three of us piled into Eric's Toyota and headed into the city.

"I can't believe it's really here," Sebastian marveled.

"Me neither," I replied.

I fretted silently. *What if the weather gets hot and he loses his vision again, or isn't careful crossing a street? He could be gone in an instant.*

"Remember, I want you to check the weather in the morning every day."

"I will," Sebastian said agreeably. He'd heard this lecture about ten million times already.

"If it's going to be in the nineties, I want you to take an Uber door to door." I couldn't help myself. I had to say it again. "I don't care if it's only three blocks, I don't want you going completely blind while you are alone in the city."

"Don't worry, Mom," he said, affectionately. He reached over the seat and patted my shoulder. "I've got this."

Dear God, I prayed silently. *Please let this be true. I don't doubt my son's capabilities, but he's only fifteen years old, severely visually impaired, and alone in the city of Chicago. He has no white cane if he goes completely blind.* I wished for the millionth time that I had the training to teach my son white-cane technique myself.

Please protect my son, I prayed again. *Don't let him be hit by a bus. Please keep the weather cool for him for these two weeks.*

Sebastian reached over the seat and I reached back; his hand in my hand.

When we arrived at the dorm for the School of the Art Institute Early College Program, it was a well-oiled machine of young adults helping teens to unload. Everyone was so welcoming. Sebastian knew his way through the building to his room from our previous rehearsal the week before. He learned his steps and turns in one trip.

After the orientation meeting, we went out to Nando's for dinner.

"I've got the Where's My Droid app all set up," Eric said. "Your mother will be watching every step you take," he joked.

"Only every other one."

"It's okay, Mom," Sebastian reassured me for the thousandth time. "Thank you for taking me to practice all these times. I know my way."

I knew it was true. We had come three days a week to walk these routes around the School of the Art Institute campus for two months; I made him lead me. Sebastian could use public transport. *It is going to be fine,* I told myself. *These two weeks will go fast, and he must practice being independent if he is going to go to college.* I had to trust his judgment and let him go.

He can manage if he stays cool. He knows how to protect himself from the heat, I thought, going through my mental checklist. *He has his water bottle. He knows to hydrate.*

"It's hard to let you fly," I said honestly. "I will be walking with you in spirit until you're home."

"Sightless flight is not so bad," Sebastian said, beaming. "I'll be fine. I'm not scared."

"You're a teenager. Teens never are."

"I used to be scared, before I knew how to find my way."

My heart lifted. He was so brave. Sebastian thought, and then smiled his stunning smile at me, his beautiful blue eyes filled his excitement and gratitude. "Thank you, Mom, for all you've done."

We dropped Sebastian off at the dorm. I gave him a hug. "Don't forget your appointment with Dr. Wister next week on Tuesday. I'll pick you up right here.

His jaw tightened and his eyes flashed. "This better be the last one. I've had enough eye exams to last me the rest of my life."

"It will be," I said. "It has to be."

Sebastian smiled. "I love you. I'll Uber if it's hot."

"I love you too."

I watched him turn and walk away. He waited at the intersection for the walk sign. Sharp teeth pierced my heart as the sign lit up. Sebastian, tall and slender, walked across the street without me. His words echoed in my head.

"I can see that there is something coming at me, but I can't identify it as a threat until it's too late."

My child, who looked completely typically sighted, was dependent on luck. No driver would know he couldn't see them coming. No passing stranger would offer him assistance. If he got hurt, no doctor would know what was wrong with him.

I watched in amazement for the billionth time as he stepped up the curb without looking down. How was this possible? I still couldn't truly imagine, but it was, and he did.

Sebastian walked, tall and straight, directly to the shiny brass doors of the dorm. He reached out his hand, as though reaching across all time and space, and put his hand on the handle. A pigeon startled in the early evening light, and I blinked as the shadow of wings brushed his shoulders. He opened the door and walked in.

Bad Actors

If enough people tell you that you're crazy, are you? I wondered. It was mid-June, and Sebastian was at the School of the Art Institute. It had been six months and we had never recovered Sebastian's face-blindness test results from Dr. Bucholz and Dr. Sturgis. I couldn't take my son to one more doctor's appointment without that piece of evidence of Sebastian's prosopagnosia. *Maybe they had forgotten about us,* I thought. It was worth a try. *I'm going to do it,* I decided. I picked up the phone.

"Good morning. Dr. Bucholz and Dr. Sturgis's office. How may I help you?"

"Hi, my name is Stephanie Duesing, and my son Sebastian was a patient of Dr. Bucholz and Dr. Sturgis. We are moving," I lied.

In my mind's eye I could see the sharp corner of that landscaping truck in my mental rearview mirror; the one I accidentally backed my brand-new Chrysler Cirrus into when Eric and I were newlyweds. I was so stressed and guilty from all the little lies I'd had to tell Eric while I was planning his surprise graduation party that I hit a truck on my way to setting up the party. The trunk of my new car was destroyed, but the landscaping truck was unscathed.

I expected to be screamed at when I told Eric what had happened, but Eric's only comment was "Are you okay?" I remembered my amazement at his calm and loving reaction. So, I was truly surprised that this lie to the receptionist came out easily and with only a little guilt. I gave myself a mental pat of encouragement and continued more boldly.

"I need to pick up Sebastian's records."

"No problem," the receptionist said. "I can have them ready for you tomorrow."

I had two doctor's appointments for myself, in the opposite direction, the next day. I wouldn't make it with the traffic, and also make my meeting at church with the other choir directors.

"That's okay, no rush. I'll pick them up on Friday, thanks."

"Okay," she said. "I'll have them ready for you then."

When I arrived at Dr. Bucholz's office, I recognized the receptionist. It was the same one with the piercings and the auburn hair.

"Hi," I greeted her casually. "I'm Stephanie Duesing. I'm here to pick up my son's records."

She looked me in the eye and said, "I'm sorry, we don't have any records for a Sebastian Duesing here."

Indignation raced up my spine and I pulled myself up to my full height. Not yelling but projecting my voice to the back of the office, I said loudly, "If I don't get my child's records, I'm going to file a lawsuit."

Without a word, the auburn-haired receptionist scuttled to the back, and a moment later, Dr. Amanda Sturgis cracked the door open and peeked through the crack. Her dark, messy bun sat precariously on the top of her head and wobbled. She winked hard at me with her right eye, and then winked again. "Yes?"

Dr. Sturgis was staring at me with unconvincing false doubtfulness. *You need some acting lessons,* I thought to myself. *I've seen much better.* I recognized her greasy face, and I knew she knew me, too.

"I'm here to get my son's records," I said firmly but politely. "I requested them in writing six months ago."

Sweat broke out across Dr. Sturgis's forehead. She pulled the door tighter around her face, her athletic body hidden. "I don't remember ever meeting you," she winked. "Or your son," she winked again. "I've never met you."

I felt fury and fear mixed together. My memory flashed. In my mind's eye I saw my mother's terrifying oily face wedged in the screen door, wanting access, wanting in. I wavered, wanting to run. Superimposed, I saw this winking deceiver's face saying KEEP OUT. The two faces merged in my mind. I stood up straighter. I had to get in. I was so afraid. I was afraid of her fear, her obvious judgment. I was afraid for my son, for his safety, his life.

I had another memory at that moment. My musical pest came to the rescue. I saw myself standing in the living room, both feet rooted to the ground, and my torso expanded with deep counterpressure. I was soaring through the aria "Hear ye, Israel" from Mendelssohn's *Elijah*.

I could feel the sound pouring through my body from the ground to the top of my head: "be not afraid, be not afraid, for I am thy God, I will strengthen thee." The F sharp major chord was brilliant as I springboarded easily from the C sharp to the high A sharp, singing "I, the Lord, will strengthen thee."

In my memory, I saw five-year-old Sebastian come flying through the front door with his friend. They stopped short and stared, silly grins on their faces.

"Mom!" Sebastian shouted.

I froze, the sound of my voice echoing around the living room and up the stairwell for six seconds as I inhaled and looked at the two little monkeys. I looked automatically to see if he was okay, but his face was flushed and excited, not teary or angry. The two of them looked at each other and giggled. I looked for Eric, who was supposed to be with him, and then heard the lawn mower in the front yard.

"What is it?" I asked. "Are you okay?"

"Mom, we could hear you across the street!" Sebastian said, his eyes bright.

"Okay?" I asked, confused. "So?"

"We could hear you across the street," he repeated, exchanging secret glances with his friend. They smiled devilishly.

I shook my head again. What was this about? "Okay... You know I have a big voice."

Sebastian giggled with his friend. "Dad's mowing the lawn."

"So?"

"We could hear you across the street over the lawn mower!"

I shook my head. "Okay?" I asked, uncertainly. I put my hand on my hip, now more confused. "This isn't the first time you've heard me sing."

"So, I came to tell you to shut the windows, but the windows are all closed."

I came back to earth in front of Dr. Dandruff, stubbornly holding the door and lying about my son's medical records. *I am going to blow the roof off this place with my voice,* I thought furiously. *If these people refuse to see me, then they will hear me, like it or not. Be not afraid.* And I was not afraid. I was not afraid of my mother, or this pissant doctor. I wanted justice, so I became justice.

I expanded my intercostal muscles, took a double back-breath inhalation, and, thanking God for giving Mendelssohn the divine inspiration to cast himself as a soprano, I thundered with all five feet, eleven and a half inches of my Wagnerian soprano glory, "YOU ARE A BAD PERSON!"

It wasn't polite. It was effective.

The sound of my speaking voice penetrated the entire office building, echoed around corners, and filled every cranny with my outrage. Dr. Sturgis crumbled like phyllo dough. She invited me into her office, winking, sweating, and shaking. She continually insisted she had never met me.

Her desk was tidy and clear, except for a manila folder with some papers lying on them. I picked up the top sheet.

"Really?" I said.

There, in Sebastian's own handwriting, were Sebastian's face-blindness test results. I picked up the test results and waved it at Dr. Sturgis, my eyes twin swords of disgust and disapproval.

Dr. Sturgis blinked both eyes so violently she looked like she was having a stroke. Her hands trembled as she gaped open-mouthed at me. *Have a grabber,* I thought.

"Do you have any idea how much you have hurt my child?" I boomed. I was not shouting, I was projecting, and I could project as far as I needed to. At that moment, I needed to project through the whole office building. I glared white-hot lasers at her winking face.

"My son is severely visually impaired," I informed her. Loudly. "He has both dorsal- and ventral-stream impairment."

Dr. Sturgis's eyes bugged out of their sockets. She blinked

hard with both eyes, and her mouth dropped open.

"Do you even know what that means?" My gaze was inescapable as Dr. Sturgis panicked and shivered.

"I will write anything you want," she gasped. "Just tell me what you want me to say."

She opened her laptop and madly started typing. She turned the screen to me repeatedly, asking "Is this okay? Is this okay?"

With enormous disgust I said, "He needs orientation and mobility services. He has topographical agnosia." If I hadn't been radiating rage, my skin would have been crawling with revulsion as Dr. Sturgis obeyed my commands. She typed furiously, and then turned the screen for my approval.

Her report said, "As prosopagnosia is not a condition that may be medically treated, adaptations to his environments is highly advised (e.g., orientation training)."

"Really?" I dripped sarcasm. "He needs help navigating because he can't recognize faces? That makes absolutely no sense!"

The office door swung open and the clinic director appeared, a large and self-important woman.

"Out of respect for our other patients, please keep your voice down," she said, authoritatively.

I was so far past the point of being intimidated, I laughed. I inhaled, intercostals expanded, and I activated my zygomatic lift to achieve the most resonance. I did not shout, I projected my cathedral-sized voice through the entire office. The pressure of the sound against the ceiling penetrated to the floor above.

"YOU HAVE SOME RESPECT FOR MY CHILD, ASSHOLE!"

It echoed satisfyingly. I had never been prouder in my life than I was right then; that moment.

The office manager paled and shut the door. Dr. Sturgis gasped like a fish, her eyes winking and blinking as I turned my fury back on the sweaty dough before me. She printed out her stupid report and shook as she signed it.

At that moment, Dr. Bucholz swept in, all fake fatherly concern and pretend innocence. He had Sebastian's file in his hand. Another bad actor, he looked like a recently bathed, male version of my mother. His expressions and mannerisms dripped insincerity, and the malevolence in his eyes flashed over his saccharine smile.

In my mind's eye, I could see my mother's greasy face superimposed over Dr. Bucholz's, the two of them twins in their callousness. I drew myself up to my full height.

"Your behavior is unprofessional and unethical," I said, jaw tight, my eyes burning suns of disapproval.

"But you left us." His voice was sugary and oh so reasonable and the lie in his eyes betrayed the unconvincing smile. He paged through the manila folder and pulled out a sheet. "You asked for your medical records."

In his hand was the letter Eric and I sent half a lifetime ago, regretfully asking for Sebastian's test results.

"No!" I took the file and the paper. "You dumped us and left my son in a severe crisis without even a referral to another therapist. This letter," I brandished it at his face, "is the letter we sent you expressing our regrets and requesting our own records. You deliberately left us to bounce from doctor to doctor without the one piece of evidence proving Sebastian needs help."

Dr. Bucholz's arrogant face went rigid, remorseless, and with no sense of guilt or personal responsibility. Behind him, Dr. Sturgis stared at Dr. Bucholz in surprise. Dr. Sturgis clearly did not know Dr. Bucholz dumped us, or that we had requested Sebastian's medical records, although Dr. Sturgis had administered the face-blindness test.

The letter we wrote requesting our records had been addressed to both of them, and Dr. Sturgis obviously didn't know anything about it, her lying about not knowing us notwithstanding. I wondered what lies Dr. Bucholz had told her and Dr. Fredericks about us. The resemblance to my own mother's behavior was unmistakable, and I made my own diagnosis mentally. I went through my list of antisocial behaviors and checked a lot of mental boxes: manipulative, deceitful, remorseless, disregard for the law and ethical standards. I stared at Dr. Bucholz with contempt.

"You are a disgrace."

I turned and left. I shook and I exulted all the way home. Later, I shared my triumph with Eric over dinner.

Eric looked at me and laughed, "As long as you didn't get arrested."

The following week Eric and I picked up Sebastian on State Street to drive out west for his final optometry appointment. I had the evidence; I had support; I had all the correct terminology. I was triumphant.

In the exam room the assistant was cheerful and nice. She was a mom herself, she told us, and she listened carefully and took great notes as we briefly went over all our findings of Sebastian's verbal visual processing.

"Sebastian looks normally sighted and is excelling academically," I said, "so we've had a really rough time getting a diagnosis."

She smiled sympathetically as I handed her the prosopagnosia test results, feeling like I was passing the Olympic flame.

"I had to go all *Xena: Warrior Princess* to get our own medical records. We had doctors actually hiding our medical records from us and pretending they didn't know us."

She laughed, "I would do the same if it was my kid."

I believed her. She was sincere.

"Doctor will be right with you," she smiled charmingly, and stepped out.

Not a moment later, Dr. Pearl Wister entered the room with a sheet of paper in her hand.

"Hi! I just got your email," she said apologetically. "I'm sorry, but I don't know anything about this or who any of these people are."

I just gaped. Sebastian's face fell. We stared at each other, wordless. Dr. Wister looked guilelessly at us. "I don't know why they sent you to me."

Unperturbed by our disappointment, Dr. Wister asked

Sebastian about how he identifies some objects around the room. There was a large cotton swab, like a giant Q-tip, and some other items. Sebastian explained his use of verbal characteristics simply and eloquently. As we waited, devastated and exhausted, Dr. Wister proceeded to give Sebastian a multi-hour, exhaustive, extremely thorough, and professional assessment for ocular blindness, which Sebastian does not have, and is not related to CVI.

Several hours later, Eric and I were finally called back to the exam room.

Dr. Wister said, "I have no expertise in this area," and that she needed "two weeks to do some research."

I emailed you two weeks ago, and you didn't respond, I thought. *You've had your two weeks.*

Out loud I said politely, "The book you need is called, *Vision and the Brain: Understanding Cerebral Visual Impairment in Children.* It's a textbook edited by Gordon Dutton." Dr. Wister looked it up on her computer as we spoke. As she looked at the blue cover of the textbook on her screen it was obvious she had never heard of it.

She asked me where Dr. Dutton was located.

"Dr. Dutton is the professor emeritus of visual sciences at Glasgow Caledonian University in Edinburgh, Scotland," I said. I was pleased that she was interested and willing to learn, even though I was more than annoyed with her lack of preparation. We wrapped up the appointment with Dr. Wister telling us she would get back to us in two weeks. I smiled and nodded.

In the car on the way home I started searching for Dr. Gordon Dutton. I couldn't find him, but I found www.cviscotland.org.

SUBJECT My son has severe CVI, we need help

Dear Professor Dutton,

My name is Stephanie Duesing and my son Sebastian is a fifteen-year-old honor student who skipped a grade and scored a perfect 150 on the verbal portion of the IQ test. In January this year we discovered he couldn't recognize himself or anyone else while going through old photos. He also has been navigating like a blind person all his life, by counting his steps and turns.

Long story short, Lukas Franck, the senior program manager at The Seeing Eye, put us in touch with Jim Deremeik, who very kindly arranged for me to take your course on CVI so that I can be a better advocate for my son. We are struggling to get a diagnosis for him here in the US.

My son has severe cerebral visual impairment. He has both dorsal and ventral stream processing dysfunction. The only visual memory he has is for words, letters, numbers, and simple shapes. He has no ability to recognize faces, places, objects or animals. He has no ability to self-orient. All of his brain scans are clear, and because of his extremely high IQ, his visual memory test scores appear to be in the average range.

However, Sebastian has to narrate constantly to himself in order to see. He uses a taxonomy of verbal descriptors to identify every ordinary day-to-day object or person he encounters all day long. For example, if he sees a backhoe he has to think "thing", then "vehicle ","construction vehicle ", and then finally "backhoe ". He goes through this process for everything he needs to identify all day long, every day.

His vision is variable and tires from use. We understand it's incredibly unusual to discover such a severe disability so late. Because of his very high IQ, Sebastian has incredible verbal compensation strategies. Genius IQ does run in my family.

We know we also missed many signs: three years of separation anxiety, fear of going to the grocery store and gymnastics class, lining toys up, and dumping toys. He was reading at age 2, had all normal developmental milestones and is not autistic.

We are struggling to get a diagnosis because his brain scans are normal and his extraordinary verbal compensation strategies make his visual memory test scores appear to fall in the average range. He's been identifying everything and everyone using verbal descriptors all his life, so the visual memory tests aren't accurate on him.

He's absolutely brilliant at math, which shouldn't be possible with average visual spatial abilities. He did score in the severely impaired range on the prosopagnosia test.

In addition to all this, Sebastian can only see a very small rectangle measuring approximately 3x2 inches while he's reading. At a distance of ten feet he has about a square yard of regular acuity. When he looks across the street, he can't see the whole house there. He says he perceives color and vague blurry shapes in the area around his rectangle of normal acuity.

I think he may possibly have simultanagnosia. When we were driving, he could see both tail lights on the truck ahead, but not the license plate between them. We are deeply concerned. Although we've only this year become aware of Seb's disability, I've always been aware of his extreme exhaustion after school. It seems to all of us, including Sebastian, that his vision tires more quickly and it's more difficult to see than it was in the past.

We are so, so in need of help. We understand there's no cure for CVI, we just need a proper diagnosis so we can access state services for orientation and mobility training. Sebastian has no ability to self-orient. He cried every day for three months telling us that he was afraid he was going to get lost when he changed schools. His therapist diagnosed him with anticipational anxiety. We are devastated for our child, that we didn't catch this sooner.

We would be so grateful for any help. Thank you for your time and consideration.

Respectfully,

Stephanie Duesing

From: Gordon Dutton:
Subject: Sebastian
Dear Ms. Duesing,

Thank you for getting in touch about your son Sebastian. I fully understand your anxieties on his behalf. Your compelling account of Sebastian's vision is indeed highly consistent with a marked form of CVI affecting both ventral and dorsal stream functions. Young people with the type of vision you describe for Sebastian, are often highly able linguistically. From my experience, what is clearly unique about your account of Sebastian, is his combination of:

Very high linguistic ability

Probable profound dorsal and ventral stream dysfunction (which he of course knows to be his normal), and

MRI imaging which has been described as normal (but could merit careful radiological review)

Of course, I understand your wish for Sebastian to be accorded a formal diagnosis. I have recently been working closely with a visual neuropsychologist in Paris, Sylvie Chokron as we share the same concept frameworks about CVI. You may find our two recent educational review publications below to be of interest:

2016 Chokron et al DCD / CVI (academic review):
http://journal.frontiersin.org/article/10.3389/fpsyg.2016.01471/full

2016 Dutton et al Posterior parietal pathology (Invited educational review for the optometry profession in the US):
http://c.ymcdn.com/sites/www.covd.org/resource/resmgr/vdr/vdr_3_1/VDR_3_1_dutton.pdf

To my knowledge she is the individual most suited to objectively characterize and thus apply a diagnostic label to Sebastian's condition, as I understand she has developed a set of salient novel investigations to do so. She and I could potentially assist you collaboratively. For my part, I would be in a position to 'brain storm' with Sylvie and yourselves to seek and to develop additional ideas that could assist Sebastian.

Notably, we have found that when those with CVI who have exceptional abilities like Sebastian, are taught to understand and have insight into their alternative normal vision, life becomes progressively easier to manage because they then become empowered to become able to devise and implement salient adaptive and compensatory strategies for themselves.

In the first instance, could I direct you to the website CVI Scotland: http://cviscotland.org

I have an iPhone and my telephone number is:
****
...if you would like to discuss these ideas further by FaceTime or telephone, perhaps later today. We are on British Summer Time (BST) at present.

With kind regards

Gordon Dutton
Emeritus Professor of Visual Science
Glasgow Caledonian University

Pacem in Terris

"The eye that sees is the I experiencing itself in what it sees."-
Frederick Franck

"In the silence of drawing,
hidden, yet visible, in each face
I see the Face of faces,
see:
that the plural of man
does not exist,
is our cruelest hallucination –
see that our Oneness is infinite differentiation,
see:
that the pattern of the universe
and mine
are not-two,
that what lives in me
is the Tao
in which all lives.
THIS IS NOT WHAT I BELIEVE
BUT WHAT MY EYES SAW ON THE WAY.
A STRANGER NO LONGER
I AM AT HOME,
BELOVED EARTH!"

-From *The Awakened Eye*, by Frederick Franck

The lavender Earl Grey tea perfumed the air sweetly as I sat at the kitchen table sorting documents and photos from the past year. It was fall of 2018, and I took a sip, inhaling and letting the lavender work its relaxing magic. The charming Allegretto movement of Mozart's Piano Concerto No.17 in G Major shimmered around me. Moby Deck stretched off to my right, now in its autumnal phase, brown and barren of flowers.

I read over the thirty-six single-spaced typed pages of

documentation of our medical journey. I'd never written a book before, and I wondered where to start. Where is the beginning of a story? I decided to begin in the middle, and I put my notes down and typed.

"Sebastian Duesing was officially identified as the only person in the world known to process his vision verbally in March of 2018."

I laughed to myself. How many others like Sebastian are walking around with no one knowing? Hundreds? Thousands? I kept typing.

"Sebastian spent six hours in the fMRI for the Harvard CVI Neuroplasticity research study, under the direction of Dr. Lotfi Merabet, where he captured Sebastian's verbal visual processing. Dr. Merabet and his team arranged to pay all our expenses to fly us out to Boston in order to participate in the research study. Although I tried to discourage him, and I told him it was totally unnecessary, Dr. Merabet himself drove across Boston to meet us at the hotel and bring us to the research study. The entire team went to extraordinary lengths to make us feel comfortable and appreciated."

I paused, remembering all the events that led up to that week in Boston. That would be another story, I decided. I kept typing.

"Sebastian is the only person in the world known to be able to choose to see or not see with his eyes wide open. When he is not narrating to himself, he has no conscious perception of sight. He can't tell if his visual world is light or dark without narration, because if he thinks either of those words, then he is seeing again."

I pulled up the fMRI image from Dr. Merabet and marveled at it, again; a stranger's neurotypically sighted control brain seeing on the left, then Sebastian's visual cortex seeing with verbal narration in the center, and finally Sebastian's brain again but without narration on the right. The stark reality of his blind/not blindness amazed me, again.

I sipped my tea and watched a squirrel ripple across Moby Deck on his way to the bird feeder, and then continued.

"Sebastian was diagnosed with CVI by Dr. Barry Kran, professor at the New England College of Optometry and director of optometrics at the New England Eye Low Vision Clinic at Perkins School for the Blind on March 27, 2018. Dr. Kran dedicated countless hours of time over several months taking history via email and through video chat. He was brilliant as well as extraordinarily kind, patient, and knowledgeable. We are and always will be grateful to him for his kindness and expertise.

Sebastian has been extensively studied. Dr. Sylvie Chokron and her team did a weeklong research study with the assistance of Dr. Gordon Dutton on Sebastian at La Fondation Rothschild in Paris, France, in September of 2017. We were treated with the utmost kindness and respect by every single person on the team. Dr. Chokron found significant brain damage using SPECT scan, which is considered safe enough for pregnant women. SPECT scans also show where brain damage is located, no matter the age of the subject. Any parts of the brain where there is no blood flow are dead tissue."

I found my teacup empty, and I rose and refilled it with freshly steaming floral nirvana. I watched the squirrel, which was now wrapped sideways around our squirrel-proof bird feeder and stuffing his face with sunflower seeds, and I smiled. I sat back down and continued typing.

"Sebastian is so severely visually impaired that according to Dr. Barry Kran, Sebastian 'would be functioning at the level of legal blindness if it were not for his extraordinary verbal compensation abilities.' Sebastian has both dorsal- and ventral-stream impairment. His dorsal-stream impairment is characterized by a difficulty spotting a distant target and visual crowding. He experiences significant visual tiring. His ventral stream is so impaired that he has no ability to recognize faces, places, objects, or biological forms. He has prosopagnosia (face blindness), object agnosia, topographical agnosia, and simultanagnosia. The only things Sebastian can recognize the way that neurotypically sighted people do are words, letters, numbers, and simple shapes.

"Sebastian has simultanagnosia. His visual fields are full, but he has only a tiny patch of acuity in the center of his visual field. When he is not too visually tired, Sebastian can usually see about three or four letters at a time when he is reading, if the font is small enough for him. He usually prefers ten-point font. The rest of his surrounding visual field is too blurry for him to make out any detail. He perceives light, color, motion, and vague blurry shapes in the area surrounding his patch of clear vision."

I paused for a moment, feeling my indignation rise as I pictured Sebastian seated in the exam chair at his eye appointments every year. My severely visually impaired son passed every vision test every year because the vision tests are flawed. Simultanagnosia is easy to test for, and so are difficulties with visual crowding. Sebastian's CVI should have been caught years ago in his eye exam. That eye care professionals refuse to provide easy assessments for common vision impairments is unconscionable and must change. I sipped my tea to calm myself, and then I continued.

"Sebastian taught himself to see with art. He memorized all the verbal characteristics of objects, animals, and people by drawing, painting, and sculpting them. Sebastian wakes up every day in a world he can't recognize, and he plays a constant guessing game of what or who is this thing, or object, or person. He is so good at guessing that he appears to be typically sighted. With the exception of words, letters, numbers, and simple shapes, Sebastian's visual memory is nonexistent. Every time he sees any other thing, it is for the very first time, every single time. His brain does not record visual images despite years of effort to learn to do so.

"When he narrates to himself, Sebastian experiences a momentary glimpse of what he's looking at. When he is narrating the characteristics of an object, he can 'get an idea of it,' he says, but it is a fleeting image with no afterimage and no retention in memory. For example, when he looks at his hand, it is the first time he has ever seen any hand, every single time. Except for moving objects such as vehicles, Sebastian's verbal visual processing is so quick that it approaches in all appearances that of neurotypical visual processing."

I sipped my tea again, now cooler, and enjoyed the spicy sweetness for a moment while I considered how to phrase the next part. Then I had it, and I continued typing.

"Sebastian is mostly unconscious of the sublingual narration as it occurs. He says it's like a background static in his brain. However, Sebastian says that when he needs to attend to auditory information such as speech, he is unable to focus well on both seeing and listening simultaneously. He can't see and listen at the same time effectively. When he needs to listen to a conversation or a lecture, he automatically turns off the narration and then he is completely blind."

I thought about having to silently recite the Declaration of Independence to myself while listening to a physics lecture on string theory. It's no wonder my son can't see and hear at the same time. I wondered what would Sebastian's life be like now if I hadn't done sign language with him when he was a baby. His language development would have been severely impaired. I exhaled hard, and then I turned back to my typing.

"Sebastian uses his blindsight to travel through the environment without conscious perception of objects and obstacles. He says his movement perception feels like a completely different sense than his verbal vision. Sebastian is incredibly independent and with the support of technology he is able to go anywhere he wants. He was accepted into the Leader Dogs for the Blind Accelerated Orientation and Mobility Program, for which we are extremely grateful, where he worked on white-cane safety skills in case of visual tiring.

"Sebastian has affective blindsight. He recognizes facial expressions even though he doesn't recognize the face itself. He says he thinks he recognizes facial expressions the same way he does everything else, with their verbal characteristics.

"Sebastian received extensive vision therapy from a highly qualified developmental optometrist, Dr. Neil Margolis, for convergence insufficiency in the fall and winter of 2018. He can locate objects in space with measurably more accuracy than he could prior to treatment, as now his stereoscopic vision and depth perception is improved.

"Cerebral/Cortical Visual Impairment is more common than ocular blindness in developed nations. Anyone at any time can acquire CVI through stroke or traumatic brain injury. We know Sebastian has CVI from birth trauma, but the concussion sophomore year worsened his simultanagnosia and difficulties with visual tiring.

"Although CVI was identified as the number-one cause of visual impairment in the developed world more than ten years ago, there are only a handful of medical professionals in the United States with any modern scientific understanding of what CVI is or how to diagnose it. In addition, the vast majority of teachers of the visually impaired (TVI) receive little to no training in how to identify, assess, teach, or assist students with CVI, although on average more than half the students in their caseloads have it.

"CVI is an entirely different disability from ocular blindness, with different causes, symptoms, and habilitative needs. Although CVI is common and often debilitating, in 2018 there was only one university training program that even required their TVI students to take coursework in CVI. That program was at the University of Massachusetts in Boston."

I sat back and sighed, remembering the educational nightmare we entered before we had even finished the medical part. So much change is needed. May this story inspire others to make a difference, so that no one else goes through what we did. I jostled the stack of papers and three photos landed on the floor beside me, one on top of the other. I inhaled sharply and almost sloshed tea on the jumble of pictures and documents.

Sebastian, skeletal, looked back at me. I could still feel his starving body as we walked gingerly, just the two of us, from the cab to the entryway of the hospital. He shuffled carefully, like an elderly man. We were in Paris, standing outside La Fondation Rothschild, just before going in to begin the research study. It was a gray day in September 2017, nine months after we discovered Sebastian's CVI.

In the photo, Sebastian's normally fair and porcelain skin was an unhealthy stark white. He looked papery and almost deathly; he was emaciated and ghostlike. He stood, frail and more than fifty pounds underweight. Almost a third of his body weight had evaporated in the four weeks since he got sick that August while we waited to take him to the research study in Paris.

I stopped him to take the photo by the La Fondation Rothschild sign. In the photo, Sebastian smiled gamely for the picture, his face skull-like and sharply defined. His vivid blue eyes burned too brightly. One tear formed in my right eye and I angrily brushed it aside. The medical malpractice from being falsely labeled crazy had not ended in June when I finally found Dr. Dutton in Scotland.

That's another story, I thought, and I took another sip of my tea. Things could be far worse for us, I knew, and far worse for Sebastian. We had so much to be thankful for. I know now that it's actually a blessing that the doctors told us he had a nine on his Apgar score when he was born. We are lucky they lied to us.

I didn't know Sebastian had a brain injury when he was a baby, and so I played musically with him as if he were healthy. I remembered the moment when I was Skyping with Gordon Dutton and I told him how my partial photographic memory for text had evaporated after Sebastian's birth.

"You had a mini-stroke," Professor Dutton said, kindly, "from the preeclampsia." His eyes were filled with compassion as I finally accepted what had happened to Sebastian, and that he had indeed painted and recognized a bird by its verbal characteristics as a toddler that day in the kitchen so long ago.

I exhaled, and then continued typing. "If I had known Sebastian had had a brain injury at birth, I would have handled him with kid gloves, afraid I would hurt him further. Because I thought he was healthy, I twirled and danced with Sebastian. I rocked and bounced him, every single day, while I sang to him.

He experienced both music and movement together throughout the day, every day. If I had known Sebastian had a brain injury, he would have experienced less movement, and his movement perception would be less developed. Sebastian has blindsight. That's why he doesn't crash into things."

I paused from my typing and had another sip of tea, enjoying the sweetness of the blend. I thought about all I had learned from Dr. Dutton's course, and I turned back to my computer.

"I believe motion vision is trainable," I typed. "It is changeable and adaptable. It's the posterior parietal lobes of the brain that are responsible for visual guidance of movement through three-dimensional space. Sebastian is living proof of the power of the arts to heal. Most kids with CVI are severely developmentally delayed. What if every child with CVI could ride a bike, or run, or play water polo? Or walk without bumping into things? With music and movement intervention in early childhood, these children can have a better quality of life."

My phone pinged again, bringing me back to the present. I glanced at it and then stared at the pile of papers and photos all over the kitchen table. My tea had gone cool, but it was still lovely as I took a sip, and my eye fell on the other photo I had jogged loose from the pile on the table. In this photo, Sebastian stands in the center of the Albrecht-Kemper Museum in St. Joseph, Missouri.

I brought both hands to my mouth and smiled behind my fingers as I bent down to see the image more clearly. In this photo, Sebastian's eyes were determined and confident. Although he was still too pale and slender, he stood proudly. His calm blue eyes bravely looked out from the photo with understanding much older than his years. Behind him, three of his paintings hung on the wall: Mimi sitting on the lid of a Starbucks cold cup, an oil painting of Kalo the macaw, and my favorite, Sebastian's Blue Figures.

The three headless figures danced joyfully through the trees, and I couldn't help smiling as I leaned back in my chair remembering the joy of Sebastian's first art exhibit. I remembered the oddness of standing in the beauty of the Albrecht-Kemper Museum in front of my seventeen-year-old son's paintings and feeling the impossibility of surviving our battle with our broken medical establishment. I felt deeply the incongruity of being surrounded by the work of artists like my son—people gifted with the ability to truly see—and the hope for the future all that talent inspired.

My phone pinged again: a new notification on Facebook. I looked and saw a comment on a CVI page; someone else searching for help. There are so many of us. The enormity of the task of writing a book yawned before me. I turned back to my keyboard and kept writing.

"The majority of developmental delays in balance, proprioception, and both fine and gross motor skills are rooted in the inner ear. Music and movement in early childhood force both sides of the brain to communicate through the corpus callosum. No other activity mimics the effects of music on the brain. There are decades of research to support that statement." In my head I pictured Cathy Mathia at my Musikgarten training class in Dallas. I could see her assured confidence as she explained all of the neuro- science behind the Musikgarten Music and Movement program.

As I typed I could see Sebastian running through the yard, chasing a soccer ball and scoring a goal. I saw him as a preschooler in swim lessons; the first volunteer to go off the diving board when he was a toddler; making accurate passes to his teammates in water polo; finely slicing a bell pepper to make his own stir fry; and of course, always painting.

I sipped my tea and then continued. "Musikgarten music and movement classes were created by Dr. Lorna Heyge and Audrey Sillick. In 1990 they met neuroscience educator Dr. Dee Coulter and were greatly influenced by her insights. Over decades they have responded through research, training, outreach, and teaching to many crisis situations in early childhood development. Their work is known across many continents.

"Dr. Coulter says, 'Rhythm may be the most important gift

you can give your child. Why? First you need to know that the highest level of brain functioning occurs in the frontal lobes. This region has its major growth spurt from birth to age six, and it must have rhythm to stimulate this growth. Rhythmic training also helps to cultivate 'motor flow' or grace by building connections between the rhythm that is heard and the movements that are paired with it."

I paused and reread my work, then smiled. Doctors would all be prescribing music to all patients of all ages if they got kickbacks, I knew. I laughed then, because music doesn't require a prescription from a doctor. I wrote my own prescription, for all my beloved CVI families. You are not alone, my people.

I typed: "Unless your doctor tells you that you can't move and sing to your baby, then you can, and you should. Every day, throughout the day, your baby needs to hear your voice, feel your movements, and move rhythmically with you through space to develop their frontal lobes."

I smiled to myself and continued typing.

"Dr. Dee Coulter says, 'We call this "sensory-motor integration" and it lays the foundation for overall coordination, for skill at sports and performance in the arts, and it leads to a joy in moving, playing, and socializing. No wonder music and movement training is now being sought out as therapy for young children with disorders ranging from ADD to ADHD, developmental delays, cerebral palsy and other motor issues, to autistic spectrum issues.'"

I stopped and sipped my cold tea, and my eye fell on the corner of Sebastian's second genetic testing panel we had done. I grimaced. I had been right about the Effexor not being safe for my son. I felt an unexpected surge of pity for Dr. Bucholz and Dr. Sturgis and the rest of our incompetent doctors. There were no safe psychotropic medications for Sebastian. I thanked God for my diligence.

I pulled the genetic test report out and set it to the side. In the process, I jostled another photo loose from the pile next to it. I picked up the photo and looked. In that picture, Sebastian sits in the fMRI at the Harvard CVI Neuroplasticity research study, surrounded by his incredible team. Sebastian smiles bravely, surrounded by Dr. Lotfi Merabet and the rest of the team, all working together with courage and decency to end this public health crisis surrounding CVI. No one who looked at the picture or read our Facebook post on the CVI Laboratory for Visual Neuroplasticity Facebook page on March 30, 2018, would ever guess the extent or seriousness of the injustice and abuse we had experienced.

I examined the photo more closely. Sebastian's eyes, so beautiful and miraculous, were changed, but only if you knew him. His once confident and cheerful outlook on the world was forged into something else; something harder and more cynical, yet determined and strong. I could hear Sebastian's voice as we talked about going to Boston for the Harvard Study. It was February, more than a year after discovering his vision impairment, and we still couldn't get help from our school despite having the excellent report from the research study in Paris and the evidence of brain damage from the SPECT scan.

"I don't want to go to Boston for the research study." Sebastian's eyes were hard. "I never want to see another doctor again." He sat up straighter and looked at me. "But I will go." His voice was steely. "I understand why it's important. It's not about me anymore. We are so far beyond that."

My heart broke and filled with pride at the same time for my son, who had so much courage and determination as a child of sixteen. Sitting alone in front of my computer in the kitchen, my eyes filled with tears as I thought of all this kid had endured, and I was filled with pride at his resilience and his concern for all the others out there with CVI. I heard his voice, strong and confident.

"I know," Sebastian said fiercely, "that I am a part of something bigger than myself."

The phone rang. I looked at the number. It was Dr. Mindy Ely, assistant professor, Low Vision and Blindness at Illinois State University. My heart rose in gratitude and affection as I remembered our first email conversations, her fascination and genuine curiosity mixed with compassion. After Sebastian and I returned from the research study in Paris, we still struggled to get a diagnosis even with the evidence of brain damage from the SPECT scans. Dr. Ely offered sincere and practical help and connected us to Dr. Kran at the Perkins School for the Blind.

"Hello, *Doctor* Ely!" I grinned as I put a little emphasis on the doctor part. "Congratulations on defending your doctoral thesis. That's a huge accomplishment."

"Thank you," she said modestly.

"How are you?"

I settled myself down on the sofa as she told me a little about what had happened since we last spoke. I sat back and enjoyed the quiet confidence in this lovely person's voice. I wondered what she looked like. Her voice was assured, intelligent, and thoughtful. Dr. Ely asked how Sebastian was doing.

"He is hanging in there," I said. "Thank you for asking. Despite everything going on, he got a 103% in AP Art History and a 5 on the exam," I bragged.

I couldn't help it. I warned you, dear reader, that I would have to brag to tell my story, so why stop now when we are almost done? How else could you know how perfectly disguised Sebastian was, from all of us?

"How weird is that?" I continued. "That a kid with almost no visual memory is a skilled artist and loves art history? Oh, and I don't know if I told you, but the wonderful Dr. Mary Morse presented Sebastian's brain scans at the Association for the Education and Rehabilitation of the Blind and Visually Impaired convention in Reno this summer. Mary has been so generous with her help, and we are so grateful to have been able to contribute something truly meaningful to the educational side of this issue as well as to the medical research."

As we chatted more, I was struck again by the tremendous kindness and true compassion for my child in Dr. Ely's voice. Her genuine concern and caring were evident as she asked about Sebastian's visual tiring.

"Sebastian is looking forward to starting braille next summer when he has time," I explained. "Although his reading comprehension is extraordinarily high, he finds the act of reading to be extremely visually exhausting."

Mindy and I talked about the online braille program available. She was so kind and supportive. She is truly a caring person, I could tell, and I wondered how she chose her field. She clearly had such deep feeling for this child she had never met.

"How did you get involved in low vision?" I asked.

"My mother lost her vision in a car accident," Mindy replied.

A shiver ran down my spine and all my attention focused on her lovely voice. I could hear the deep love and sadness for her mom's pain and suffering as she relived the memory. Her voice was filled with grief and regret as she told me her story. I said a silent prayer of thanks that God brought this brilliant and compassionate woman into our path.

I exhaled and sat back on the sofa. "I am so sorry," I said. Sorry is such a useless word sometimes. I felt my thoughts spiraling down my long chain of memories and I brought myself back to the present with effort. I tried again. "That must have been awful." I was totally failing to express my condolences, I knew. I vacillated for a moment, and then I decided to tell her before I made things any worse.

"You know, my mother went blind after a car accident as well."

"What happened?" Dr. Ely asked, genuinely curious.

"She flipped her car on the expressway and was in a body cast for a year. A tiny piece of cartilage blocked the artery that fed the optic nerve to her left eye."

"That would do it," Dr. Ely agreed. Then thoughtfully, she said, "You know, you are the only other person I have ever met who knew someone who lost her vision in a car accident."

"Me, too!" I agreed, my eyes stinging. Hastily I changed the subject. "You must have gotten my email," I began apologetically. "I truly am so sorry about the longitudinal research study we talked about. I know you have put in a tremendous amount of work on the proposal, and I feel terrible about disappointing you.

Sebastian is just sick of having his whole life revolve around his vision. He's just a kid. He wants to make his art and move on."

"Oh, don't worry about it at all. That's actually not what I called to talk about," Dr. Ely said, all kind understanding and excitement. I could hear the anticipation in her voice.

I put my tea down and leaned forward.

"What's up?"

Acknowledgements

Frederick Franck says:

> "I know artists whose medium is life itself, and who express the inexpressible without brush, paint, chisel or guitar. They neither paint nor dance. Their medium is Being. Whatever their hand touches has increased life.... They are the artists of being alive."

Thank you to my husband and best friend, Eric. I count the day I met Eric as the day my life began. Eric has supported every whim of mine for more than a quarter century, and I couldn't have written this book without his love and support.

The first people who offered us concrete help were my childhood friend and inspiration, Dr. Patricia Kelly, occupational therapist, and Joe Cioffi, CEO of ClickandGo Wayfinding. You provided essential information about IEPs and services for the visually impaired, for which we will always be extremely grateful.

This story would have had a very different ending without Pauline Cerf Alexander at the Seeing Eye. Thank you for trusting your instincts. Your compassionate heart heard my cry for help and connected us to Lukas Franck.

Lukas Franck, senior consultant at the Seeing Eye. I can't draw well, and to illustrate both the size of your heart and my gratitude for it in words is an even more provoking problem. Thank you for the dual gifts of recognition and action, one human being to another.

We extend our deepest gratitude to the Seeing Eye guide dog organization for the continuous support and caring for Sebastian and for all people with blindness and visual impairments. We are profoundly thankful for your intervention in Sebastian's case.

Lukas and the Seeing Eye brought our dire situation to the attention of Gala Brooks, and to Jim Deremeik, the head of rehabilitation at the Johns Hopkins Eye Institute, for whose compassion and ingenious generosity we will always be deeply grateful.

Another organization very dear to our hearts is the Chicago Lighthouse, especially the technology team, which was headed by Tom Perski, the senior vice president of rehabilitation; Luke Scriven, assistive technology manager; and Eric Cromey, the desktop computer and adaptive technology specialist. Your willingness to help a child with an as-yet-unknown diagnosis and your unquestioning support for individuals with CVI is a model for all others and we are deeply grateful for the kindness and support.

Char Laursen, MS CCC SLP, speech language pathologist, was instrumental in helping to confirm Sebastian's object agnosia. Your brilliant questioning and factual knowledge of CVI made an enormous difference in our lives, and your kindness to us in a challenging time will never be forgotten. We also thank Kaitlyn Peters for her outstanding services in occupational therapy. Your professionalism and deep compassion will never be forgotten.

It was Helen St. Clair Tracy's enormous love and devotion to her son that lead her to create the CVI Scotland website, which is now considered one of the best sources for factual information about CVI. Without this resource, and her kind assistance, I would never have found Dr. Dutton. Thank you for connecting us with him. We also thank Janet Harwood for her work with the CVI Society Facebook page.

Dr. Gordon N. Dutton, pediatric ophthalmologist and professor emeritus of visual sciences at Glasgow Caledonian University in Scotland. You, dear sir, I draw with inadequate words of admiration for your contributions to the world of visual perception. If I had the ability, my thanks to you would be a colossal canvas, deep with the bright pigment of provable science, the form of brilliant publications, and the scopic line of patients and outright strangers like us whose lives you have helped so immensely. Thank you for believing me and for having the heart and insight to ask your patient what he saw those many years ago: "Two black holes in your head, of course!" For months, doctors demanded that we prove Sebastian couldn't see. Not a single one of them ever asked him what he could see. Your perspicacity, sensitivity, and sagacity I attempt to draw with words, but with inadequacy for our gratitude. The artistry of your life's work saved my son's. There are no words of thanks for that.

Dr. Sylvie Chokron, director of research, Department of Functional Vision and Cognition, at La Fondation Rothschild, in Paris, France: You sculpted miracles out of emergencies and arranging that SPECT scan was a heroic feat by itself. Thank you for your brilliant research contributions to the CVI field, and for the extraordinary patience, compassion, and understanding you showed to all of us.

Dr. Fiora Martinelli, neuropsychologist at le Centre Hospitalier de Castelluccio – Pôle de Psychiatrie Infanto-juvénile, Paris area, France. Thank you for your outstanding neuropsychiatric visual-spatial assessment of Sebastian, and for your grace, humor, and kindness during the process.

Lucy, our translator. Thank you for being Sebastian's linguistic superhero. You are and were an inspiration.

Dr. Barry Kran, professor, New England College of Optometry, and optometric director of the New England Eye Low Vision Clinic at the Perkins School for the Blind. You are a monument of humility and decency. Your extraordinary dedication to your patients is remarkable, but it was your intense curiosity and willingness to learn from us that makes you so exceptional. Thank you especially for your immense compassion for our traumatized family. We will always be grateful to you for your help in bringing Sebastian's visual impairment to light, and your continued advocacy efforts on behalf of all people with CVI.

Dr. Lotfi Merabet, director of the Harvard CVI Neuroplasticity research study, associate scientist at Massachusetts Eye and Ear, and associate professor of ophthalmology at Harvard Medical School. You are a brilliant man of uncommon graciousness and good manners. We were honored to be able to contribute to the understanding of CVI and visual neuroplasticity, and your efforts on our behalf made it financially possible. We are so grateful to you and to the rest of your team for arranging for the airfare and hotel accommodations, without which our emotionally and financially devastated family could not have come and participated in this crucial work. Thank you for caring about Sebastian and all people with CVI.

The Harvard CVI Neuroplasticity research study is indeed a team effort. Dr. Corinna Bauer, Dr. Christopher Bennett, Andy Ellison, and Emma Bailin worked tirelessly to compact the research study into a two-day effort. Dr. Bauer is an outspoken advocate for understanding the scientific research and medical realities of CVI, and Dr. Bennett was the creator of the ingenious virtual-reality eye-movement-tracking software that was used to capture Sebastian's verbal visual processing in the fMRI. We are so grateful to all of you for your commitment to this important work.

Finding Dr. Mindy Ely, associate professor of low vision at Illinois State University, was a stroke of luck. She immediately brought in Susan Sullivan, the CVI project leader at the American Printing House for the Blind, and Dr. Mary T. Morse, special education consultant and certified teacher of the visually impaired. All three of you touched our lives immensely. Special thanks to Dr. Ely for allowing me to share part of your story in this book, and to Dr. Mary Morse for your incredible generosity. Dr. Morse kindly volunteered to waive her consulting fee when she saw that our medical nightmare was immediately followed by educational malpractice, which will be a whole other book. We are forever grateful to you three ladies and feel deeply blessed to have you in our lives.

Dr. Neil Margolis, O.D., FCOVD, developmental optometrist and vision therapy specialist, provided Sebastian with outstanding vision therapy for convergence insufficiency, and Gretchen, his assistant, made each session of vision therapy effective and enjoyable. Thank you both for the quality care and your commitment to helping those with CVI.

Our deepest gratitude goes to Leader Dogs for the Blind, which flew Sebastian out to Michigan, all expenses paid, for a lifesaving week at their orientation and mobility intensive camp in April 2019. Special thanks go to Erica Ihrke, extended services manager and certified orientation and mobility specialist; Sarah Osaer, extended services coordinator; and Leslie Hoskins, certified orientation and mobility specialist for all their kindness, deep expertise, and flexibility. Sebastian's experience at Leader Dogs was life-changing, and we can never express our thanks adequately for the outstanding services and the caring kindness to our son.

I am so grateful to the creators of Musikgarten, Lorna Heyge and Audrey Sillick, and to Dr. Dee Coulter, neuroscience educator, for their immense gift to our family and the world. I would not know of their work without my friends and mentors, Caryn Borgetti, Leilani Miranda, and Cathy Mathia. Thank you all for your inspiration.

To Brett Knappe, the executive director of the Albrecht-Kemper Museum in St. Joseph, Missouri, and Megan Benitz, registrar and exhibitions manager. Thank you for the incredible kindness and support for Sebastian and our efforts to bring attention to the public health crisis surrounding CVI.

We extend our gratitude to Karla Cossa, and to all of Sebastian's art teachers who have been so supportive and inspirational to him. Kathryn Steinbring, you touched Sebastian's life forever with your endless support. Sebastian will always appreciate your guidance and mentorship so much. Deepest thanks go to Donald Dvorak, Mollie Bozarth, and Donna Davis as well. We thank the faculty and staff at the School of the Art Institute of Chicago, especially Valerie St. Germaine and Asia Mitchell. Sebastian is especially grateful for his Core Studio teachers, Loretta Bourque, Troy Briggs, Lisa Gaedike, and Trevor Hormel.

My friends Ken Denson, Katie Johnson, Maggie Bergren, Dagbjort Andresdottir, Jennifer Novak Carroll, Julie K. Jessen,

Tatiana Calhamer, Carol Reinheimer, Tracy Wilks, and Susan Czechowicz saw me through an event that ravaged our family. Ken had, by some amazing insight, the ability to know exactly when I needed to talk to someone badly. He just kept on checking in on me, and I think he may have saved my sanity in the process. Thank you all, my friends.

I will be working on healing my trauma for the rest of my life, but I could never have begun the process without the skill and compassion of my therapist, the wonderful and brilliant Christina Cal-Cosky, LCSW. Thank you for your insight, compassion, and persistence.

We send special thanks to Sebastian's friends, especially Natalí Craff-Bedoya. You were there when Sebastian needed a friend most, had thousands of laughs with him, and best of all, shared your chickens with him. We also thank Eun Lee, for all the Target trips and late-night worm monster hours. Sebastian says, "You are awesome. You are going to do great things. I hope we do some of them together." Sebastian also is grateful to his friends Tirzah Lawson, Ronan Shaner, Elliot Casey, Iza S., Abi, and Damien. He thanks you for the D&D sessions, bastard hours, and inside jokes. We are all grateful Sebastian has such a kind, funny, and talented group of friends.

Our thanks would not be complete without recognizing Marcus. We could not ask for a more loving, caring, and talented partner for our son. We are blessed to have you in our lives. Sebastian says, "You were there through everything and that means the world to me. I can't imagine how all this would have gone without you. Thank you for always being there."

My friends and colleagues at Our Saviour's Lutheran Church deserve special mention; especially Lynn Panosh, former director of worship and the arts, Terry Thompson, and Sue Bergren. Sue, organist and carillonneur extraordinaire, flew in with healing herbal teas from her private apothecary like a suburban fairy godmother when I was most in need. Your care and friendship mean so much. Keith and Robyn Carlson were also hugely helpful and supportive.

We are blessed to have many outstanding doctors who provided care for other conditions with great compassion and skill during an extraordinarily challenging time. They include Dr. Steven Neuberger, Dr. Michael Malandra, Dr. Alexandru Barboi, Dr. Matthew Bueche, Dr. Ashley Stoecker, and Kelly Owens, PA-C. There are amazing, kind, and generous people in this world, and these health care providers are some of the very best of them.

I wouldn't be here without the best of teachers. I thank all of them, including Penny Ellsworth, who I used to wish was my mother when I was in sixth grade. Your lessons in philosophy and logic came in handy. I also thank Bill McKay, John Sutco, Bob Boyd, Maria Lagios, Adrienne Cury, Linda Gillum, Jenny Moreau, Kurt Naebig, and John Hildreth.

It was obvious to me, as a first-time author, that I needed some professional assistance to make this story as strong as it could be. Justine Duhr at WriteByNight paired me with the wise and kind Robert McDowell for a manuscript review. Robert's gentle humor and Socratic teaching methods helped me to untangle issues with character development, and he constantly encouraged me. I am so grateful to have him as an editor and friend. Thank you, Robert, for guiding me through this process.

Our entire family is enormously grateful to my publisher, Atmosphere Press, and to Nick Courtright for his dedication to the art of publication and his compassion to our family in a time of great need. Nick made miracles happen and did it with enormous professionalism and courtesy. We are so grateful to you for your caring and kindness. Thank you for all you have done to make this book a reality.

All stories are a circle, and ours begins and ends with my son. Sebastian's soaring, almost-sightless flight through our imperfect sanctuary is almost done, and he will roost in higher aeries with extra eyes to see his journey. Sleek black Corvidae and piebald pigeons will be the feathered lashes of his city fenestrations. I am honored to be his mother; he is a man of grace and sarcastic humor, whose painted feathers charm and spell my undeveloped eye without exaggeration. What are his characteristics? Artist and astronomer, skier and philosopher. My insufficient scribble is a pale infatuation with the truth. His thaumaturgical potentiality occupied my heart and blinded my senses. He is himself, and I love him in his totality. I thank him for all joy, redemption, and forgiveness.

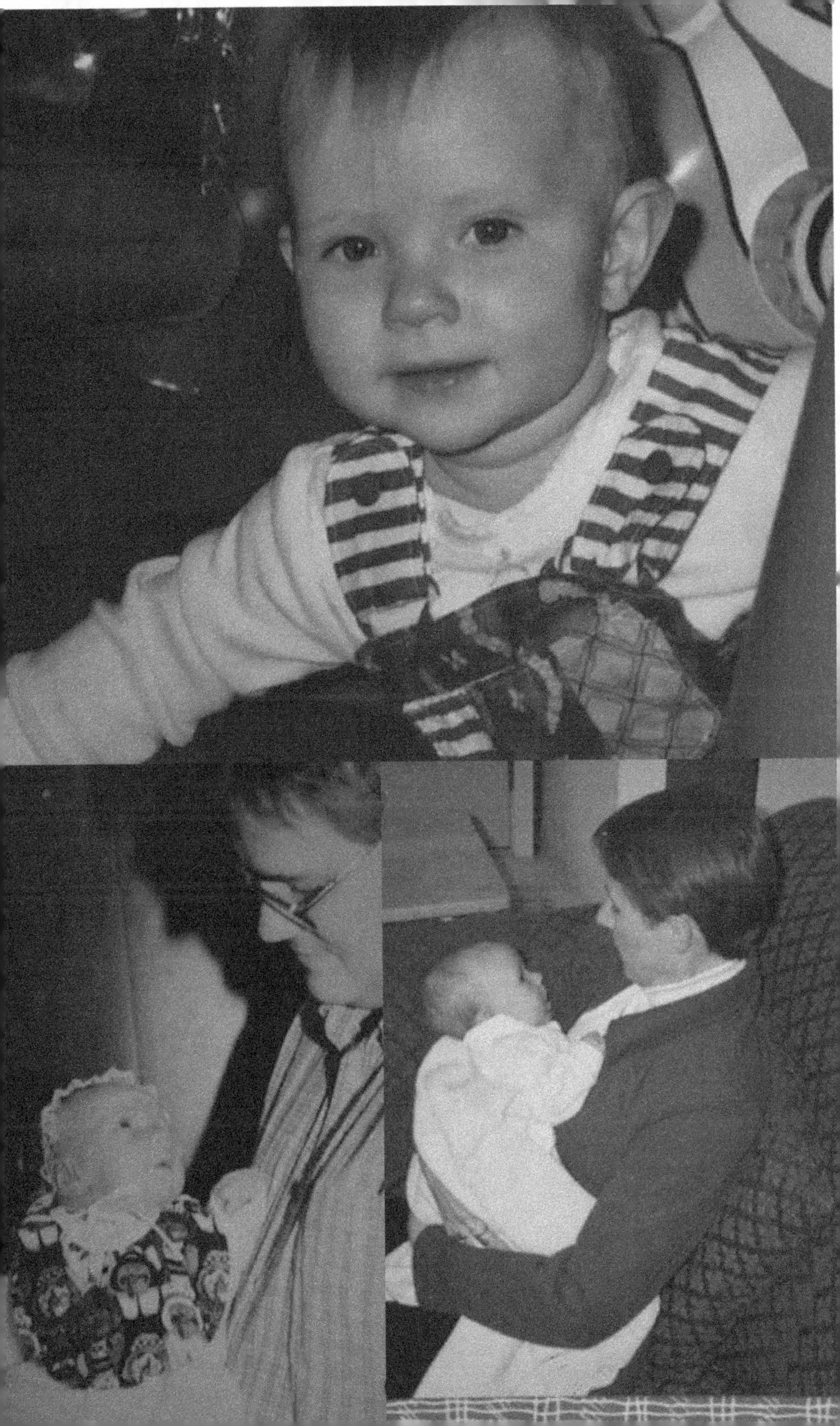

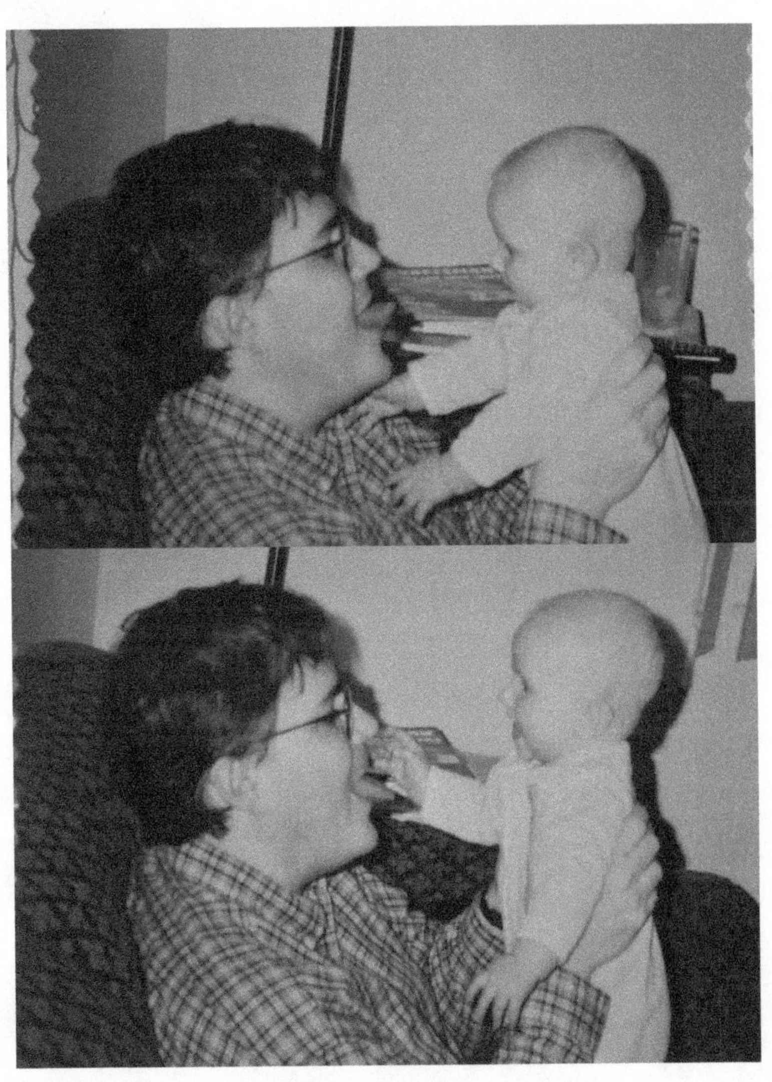

Selected Bibliography

Coulter, D. (2008)
Musikgarten Delivers! Partnering with Parents. Greensboro, N.C.: Musikgarten / Music Matters.

Franck, F. (1980)
The Awakened Eye. London, UK: Wildwood House, Ltd.

Franck, F. (2004) Editor.
The Buddha Eye. Bloomington, IN: World Wisdom, Inc.

Franck, F. (2005)
Messenger of the Heart: The Book of Angelus Silesius. Bloomington, IN: World Wisdom, Inc.

Franck, F. (2011)
Pacem in Terris: A Love Story. New Palz, NY: Codhill Press

Franck, F. (1973)
The Zen of Seeing: Seeing/Drawing as Meditation. New York: Vintage Books - Random House.

Franck, F. (1979)
Everyone: The Timeless Myth of "Everyman" Reborn. Sydney, Australia: Bookwise (Australia) Pty Ltd.

Heyge, L. L. and Sillick, A. (2007)
Music and Movement: Family Music for Babies Teacher's Guide and Resource Materials. Greensboro, NC.: Musikgarten / Music Matters.

Heyge, L. L. and Sillick, A. (2003)
*Musikgarten Music and Movement Series Family Music: Volume I, Sing with Me * Dance With Me, Teacher's Guide and Resource Materials*. Greensboro, NC.: Musikgarten / Music Matters.

Heyge, L. L. and Sillick, A. (2003)
*Musikgarten Music and Movement Series Family Music: Volume II, Play with Me * Clap with Me, Teacher's Guide and Resource Materials*. Greensboro, NC.: Musikgarten / Music Matters.

Heyge, L. L. and Sillick, A. (2007)
Music and Movement The Cycle of Seasons: A Musical

Celebration of the Year for Young Children, Teacher's Guide and Resource Materials. Greensboro, N.C.: Musikgarten / Music Matters.

Heyge, L. L. and Sillick, A. (2010)
Music Makers: At Home in the World, Teacher's Guide and Resource Materials. Greensboro, N. C.: Musikgarten / Music Matters.

Heyge, L. L. and Sillick, A. (2015)
Music Makers Around the World, Teacher's Guide and Resource Materials. Greensboro, N. C.: Musikgarten / Music Matters.

Heyge, L. L. and Hallquist, M. (2006)
Musikgarten All Together Now, A Guide to Teaching Mixed Ages. Greensboro, N.C.: Musikgarten / Music Matters.

Hundley, R. "The Astronomers."
Eight Songs (voice and piano). New York: Boosey & Hawkes, 1989.

Luecke, A. H. and Dutton, G. N. Editors. (2015)
Vision and the Brain: Understanding Cerebral Visual Impairment in Children. New York, NY. AFB Press.

Walker, G., "I Will Be Earth"
Mornings Innocent, from text by Swenson, M. St. Louis, MO: E.C. Schirmer Publishing, 1993.

All Scripture quotations, unless otherwise indicated, are taken from the Holy Bible, New International Version, NIV.

About Atmosphere Press

Atmosphere Press is an independent, full-service publisher for excellent books in all genres and for all audiences. Learn more about what we do at atmospherepress.com.

We encourage you to check out some of Atmosphere's latest nonfiction releases, which are available at Amazon.com and via order from your local bookstore:

Rags to Rags, nonfiction by Ellie Guzman
The Naked Truth, nonfiction by Harry Trotter
Heat in the Vegas Night, nonfiction by Jerry Reedy
Evelio's Garden, nonfiction by Sandra Shaw Homer
Difficulty Swallowing, essays by Kym Cunningham
A User Guide to the Unconscious Mind, nonfiction by Tatiana Lukyanova
To the Next Step: Your Guide from High School and College to The Real World, nonfiction by Kyle Grappone
Breathing New Life: Finding Happiness after Tragedy, nonfiction by Bunny Leach
Channel: How to be a Clear Channel for Inspiration by Listening, Enjoying, and Trusting Your Intuition, nonfiction by Jessica Ang
Love Your Vibe: Using the Power of Sound to Take Command of Your Life, nonfiction by Matt Omo
Leaving the Ladder: An Ex-Corporate Girl's Guide from the Rat Race to Fulfilment, nonfiction by Lynda Bayada
Letting Nicki Go: A Mother's Journey through Her Daughter's Cancer, nonfiction by Bunny Leach

About the Author

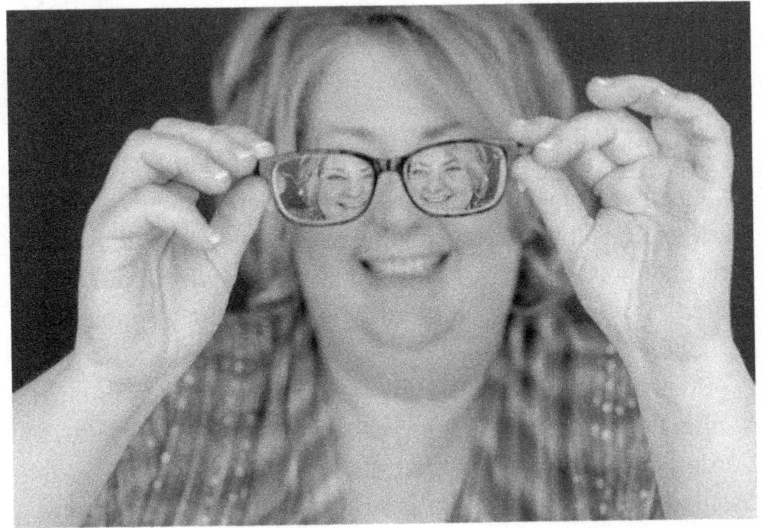

Stephanie Duesing discovered, documented, and diagnosed the first known case of neuroplastic verbal visual processing in her genius artist son, Sebastian. A music teacher with many years of experience teaching people of all ages to sing, Stephanie's hobbies include stress eating, cooking, and sneaking animals into the house when her husband isn't looking. So far, she's managed one Pomeranian, nine guinea pigs, two parakeets, a dusky conure named Mimi, and a goldfish that was too big to flush. She is not divorced.

When she's not cleaning cages, Stephanie is a self-taught expert in the science of visual neuroplasticity, and also homemade marshmallows. By necessity, she is bringing awareness to the public health crisis surrounding the diagnosis, education, and habilitation of people with neurological visual impairments. She hopes to do so with some much-needed laughter. Through her writing and speaking, Stephanie brings hope to the thousands of parents of children affected by CVI that they too can take steps to improve outcomes for their children.

Stephanie is the previous author of thousands of worksheets on the quarter note. She dedicated many minutes of her life to clearing up the conundrum of rhythmic subdivision, mostly for her own sake, and then graduated to writing sincere but unloved children's church choir newsletters. There, she solicited money for the spring musical T-shirts and reminded everyone to please take their kindergarteners to the bathroom. From there, she advanced to a position writing magazine-length newsletters for her Musikgarten families extolling the neuroscience of music in early childhood. Knowing that her newsletters were immediately stuffed into diaper bags with juice boxes and dirty nappies only encouraged her.

Stephanie is also the author of hundreds of pages of emails documenting her son's unique verbal visual processing with: Dr. Gordon Dutton, professor emeritus of visual sciences at Glasgow Caledonian University in Glasgow, Scotland; Dr. Sylvie Chokron, director of research at La Fondation Rothschild in Paris, France; Dr. Barry Kran, the head of optometrics at the New England Eye Low Vision Clinic at the Perkins School for the Blind; and Dr. Mindy Ely, associate professor of low vision at Illinois State University. These conversations are an important part of the history of understanding the only known case of verbal visual processing in the world, and are historically important in scientific, medical, and educational communities that interact with people with neurological visual impairments.

Stephanie lives at home with her beloved husband and her favorite child. A survivor of life-threatening child abuse, she is an unapologetic advocate for all victims of abuse, animal and human.

About the Artist

Sebastian Duesing is an artist/art history enthusiast/bird enthusiast currently studying for a BFA in art studio, with an art history thesis. His studio interests include painting, drawing, bookbinding, ceramics, installation, and large-scale sculpture. Sebastian had three artworks on exhibit at the Albrecht-Kemper Museum in St. Joseph, Missouri, at the age of seventeen. He recently received the Presidential Award and scholarship to the School of the Art Institute in Chicago. He aspires to become a museum curator and keep chickens. You can follow his latest projects @soaptoaster on Instagram, and purchase his art at www.sebastianduesing.com.

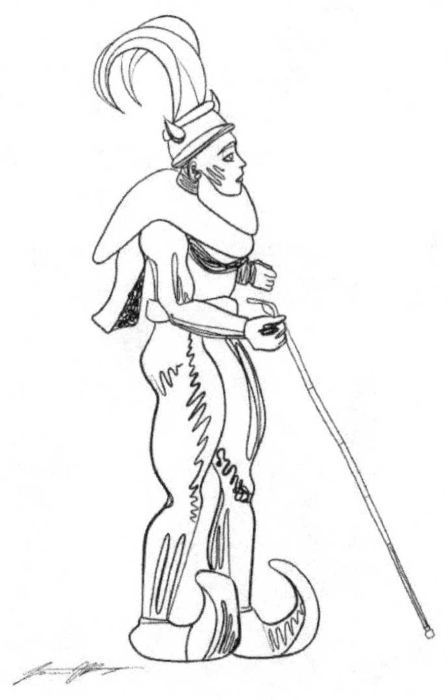

About the Author